Dasgupta's

Recent Advances in
Obstetrics and Gynecology

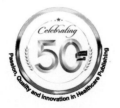

Dasgupta's
Recent Advances in
Obstetrics and Gynecology

Volume 11

Editors

Nandita Palshetkar MD FCPS FICOG FRCOG (UK)
President, FOGSI 2019
President, IAGE (2017–18)
Chairperson, MSR (2017–18)
President, AMOGS (2018–20)
Scientific Director, Bloom IVF
Professor, Department of Obstetrics and Gynecology
Dr DY Patil Medical College Hospital and Research Center
Navi Mumbai, Maharashtra, India

Pratik Tambe MD FICOG
ART Consultant and Gynecology Endoscopic Surgeon
Chairperson, FOGSI Endocrinology Committee (2017–19)
Managing Council Member, MOGS
Managing Council Member, IAGE, MSR, AMC (2015–18)

Rohan Palshetkar MS (Obs/Gyn) FRM
ART Consultant and Endoscopic Surgeon
Associate Professor
Unit Head DY Patil Bloom IVF
Navi Mumbai, Maharashtra, India

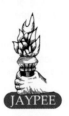

JAYPEE

JAYPEE BROTHERS MEDICAL PUBLISHERS
The Health Sciences Publisher
New Delhi | London

Jaypee Brothers Medical Publishers (P) Ltd

Headquarters
Jaypee Brothers Medical Publishers (P) Ltd
4838/24, Ansari Road, Daryaganj
New Delhi 110 002, India
Phone: +91-11-43574357
Fax: +91-11-43574314
E-mail: jaypee@jaypeebrothers.com

Overseas Office
JP Medical Ltd
83 Victoria Street, London
SW1H 0HW (UK)
Phone: +44 20 3170 8910
Fax: +44 (0)20 3008 6180
E-mail: info@jpmedpub.com

Website: www.jaypeebrothers.com
Website: www.jaypeedigital.com

© 2020, Jaypee Brothers Medical Publishers

Inquiries for bulk sales may be solicited at: jaypee@jaypeebrothers.com

Dasgupta's Recent Advances in Obstetrics and Gynecology (Volume 11)

First Edition: **2020**

ISBN 978-93-89776-53-9

Printed at: Samrat Offset Pvt. Ltd.

Dedicated to
Our teachers, mentors, and patients

Contributors

Ameya Purandare
MBBS MD (Obs and Gyne) DNBE FCPS DGO
DFP FICMCH MNAMS FICOG
Consultant Gynecologist
Sir HN Reliance Foundation Hospital
and Research Center
Mumbai, Maharashtra, India

Aswath Kumar MD FICOG Diploma in
Advanced Laparoscopy (France) Diploma
in Laparoscopic Management of Advanced
Endometriosis (Austria)
Fellow (Gynec-Oncology)
The Gujarat Cancer and Research
Institute, Ahmedabad, Gujarat (GCRI)
Professor, Department of Gynecology
Jubilee Mission Medical College
Thrissur, Kerala, India
FOGSI Quiz Committee Chairperson
(2012–2015)
Vice President, FOGSI, 2019
Vice President, KFOG, 2017

Chaithra TM
MBBS, MS (O&G), Fellowship
(Gynaec Endoscopy, Rajiv Gandhi University
of Health Sciences, Bangalore)
Consultant, Department of Obstetrics
and Gynecology
Lourdes Hospital, Kochi, Kerala, India

Hrishikesh Pai
MD FCPS FICOG MSc (USA) FRCOG
Scientific Director, Bloom IVF
Secretary General, FOGSI 2015-17
Gynecologist and Head of IVF Unit
Lilavati Hospital
Mumbai, Maharashtra, India

Jiteeka Thakkar MBBS DGO DFP
Consultant Obstetrician and
Gynecologist and Infertility Specialist
Kedia Nursing Home
Consultant Bloom IVF, Lilavati Hospital
Mumbai, Maharashtra, India

Karishma Kirti MBBS MS
HBNI Fellow
Tata Memorial Hospital
Mumbai, Maharashtra, India

Mohan A Gadam MD DGO FCPS
Consultant Obstetrician and
Gynecologist
Nanavati Superspecialty Hospital
Mumbai, Maharashtra, India

N Sanjeeva Reddy MD DGO
Professor and Head
Department of Reproductive Medicine
and Surgery
Sri Ramachandra Medical College and
Research Institute
Chennai, Tamil Nadu, India

Nandita Palshetkar
MD FCPS FICOG FRCOG (UK)
President, FOGSI 2019
President, IAGE (2017–18)
Chairperson, MSR (2017–18)
President, AMOGS (2018–20)
Scientific Director, Bloom IVF
Professor
Department of Obstetrics and
Gynecology
Dr DY Patil Medical College Hospital
and Research Center
Navi Mumbai, Maharashtra, India

Nita S Nair MD
Professor and Consultant, Department
of Obstetrics and Gynecology
Tata Memorial Center
Mumbai, Maharashtra, India

Pankaj Sarode MD
Obstetrician, Gynecologist and Infertility
Specialist
Pimple Nilakh
Pune, Maharashtra, India

Parag Biniwale MD FICOG FICMCH
Consultant Obstetrician and
Gynecologist, Cloudnine Hospital
Secretary, ICOG
Pune, Maharashtra, India

Pratap Kumar MD DGO FICS FICOG
Professor, Department of Obstetrics and
Gynecology, Kasturba Medical College
Manipal Assisted Reproductive Center
(MARC)
Manipal Academy of Higher Education
(MAHE), Manipal, Karnataka, India

Pratik Tambe MD FICOG
ART Consultant and Gynecology-
Endoscopic Surgeon
Chairperson, FOGSI Endocrinology
Committee (2017–2019)
Managing Council Member, MOGS
Managing Council Member
MSR, AMC, IAGE

Radha Vembu
MBBS DGO DNB MNAMS FICS FICOG PhD
Associate Professor
Departmentt of Reproductive Medicine
and Surgery
Sri Ramachandra Institute of Higher
Education and Research
Chennai, Tamil Nadu, India

Rajkumar H Shah MD FCPS FICS
Consultant Gynecologist and
Obstetrician, Nanavati Superspecialty
Hospital Mumbai, Maharashtra, India

Rohan Palshetkar MS(Obs/Gyne) FRM
ART Consultant and Endoscopic Surgeon
Associate Professor
DY Patil Medical College
Unit Head, DY Patil Bloom IVF
Navi Mumbai, Maharashtra, India

Rushika Mistry
MSc Life Science (Applied Medicine)
Senior Embryologist
Bloom IVF Lilavati Hospital
Mumbai, Maharashtra, India

S Shanthakumari
MD DNB FICOG FRCPI (Ireland)FRCOG (UK)
Chairperson, ICOG, 2018
Consultant, Yashoda Hospital
Hyderabad, Telangana, India
ICOG Secretary (2015–2017)
Member, FIGO Working Group
(on Violence Against Women)
Vice President, FOGSI 2013

Sandip Datta Roy
MBBS MS (OB/GYN) FICMCH FICS FMIS
(Fellowship in Gynecological Endoscopy)
Consultant Gynecologist
Laparoscopic Surgeon and Infertility
Specialist
Gem Hospital and Research Center
Thrissur, Kerala, India

Shraddha Agarwal MBBS DGO
Consultant
Department of Obstetrics and
Gynecology
KC Hospital
President
Palwal Obstetrics and Gynecology
Society
Palwal, Haryana, India

Vineet Mishra
MBBS MD (Obs and Gyne) PhD (Oxidative
Stress in Female Reproductive Life Span)
Obstetrician and Gynecologist
Dr HL Trivedi Institute of
Transplantation Sciences (IKDRC-ITS)
Civil Hospital Campus
Ahmedabad, Gujarat, India

Preface

Respected colleagues and dear friends,

It is with immense pride that we bring to you this 11th volume of *Dasgupta's Recent Advances in Obstetrics and Gynecology*. This series seeks to address a much felt lacuna in postgraduate teaching.

As you may be aware, postgraduate teaching in India is classically behind the curve as compared to our Western counterparts. While on paper, there are bedside clinics, grand rounds, hands on surgical experience, departmental lectures and journal clubs; often these are few and far between. The Western concept of protected learning time for postgraduates and residents unfortunately does not exist in India.

> *The only limit to our realization of tomorrow will be our doubts of today. Let us move forward with strong and active faith*
> *—Franklin D Roosevelt*

Often students only receive a short period of study leave prior to the examinations during which, precious time is lost scouring for resources and locating updated guidelines, research papers, and evidence on topics of thematic interest. Hence, we felt that we should address this paucity with this textbook series which aims to unite senior, respected, and stalwart postgraduate teachers from all over India who have been mentors and guides to generations of students. Each of the chapters in this book is a crash course on the subject and will serve the reader well by focusing on traditional concepts as well as the most modern updated evidence on the issues at hand.

We hope that this book will be a useful compendium for postgraduate students and readers who wish to keep themselves updated with the latest evidence on the topics we have covered. The chapters have been carefully chosen keeping in mind the current proceedings at national and international meetings while keeping the language used simple, easy to understand, and concise.

We welcome your feedback on this volume and suggestions for future topics which you may wish to see covered.

Yours sincerely,

Nandita Palshetkar
Pratik Tambe
Rohan Palshetkar

Acknowledgments

The editors would like to acknowledge the efforts of all the authors and contributors in the preparation of the manuscript, revision of their chapters, and for reverting back to us within the deadlines.

We also wish to place on record our gratitude to our publishers M/s Jaypee Brothers Medical Publishers (P) Ltd. New Delhi, India and their team led by Sabarish Menon (Mumbai Branch) and Kritika Dua (Senior Development Editor) for their kind cooperation during the layout, design, and printing process.

Contents

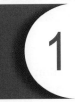
Preterm Labor

Pratap Kumar ■

■ LEARNING OBJECTIVES

- Understand importance of preterm birth
- Identify who is at risk and review prevention options
- Understand prompt management of initial presentation
- Review management of preterm premature rupture of membranes
- Management of preterm labor.

■ MAJOR CAUSES OF PRETERM BIRTH[1]

- Preterm premature rupture of membranes (PPROM): 20–30%.
- Iatrogenic:
  - Maternal indications (preeclampsia, diabetes, prior classical cesarean delivery)
  - Fetal indications (nonreassuring fetal testing, intrauterine fetal growth restriction): 20%.
- Spontaneous (unexplained preterm labor: 25–30%.
- Infection/inflammation: 20–25%.

The major causes of preterm birth (PTB) have been shown in **Figure 1**.

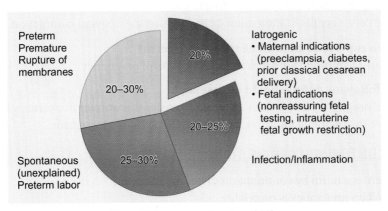

Fig. 1: Major causes of preterm birth.

▓ LATEST INTERNATIONAL GUIDELINES

There are several International guidelines such as the European Association of Perinatal Medicine 2017, Western Australian PTB prevention key initiative 2017, French clinical practice guidelines 2016, NICE guideline 2015, FIGO 2015, StratOG by RCOG 2014, ACOG 2012, SOGC 2008.

All the guidelines have uniformly stressed upon the use of progesterone as an alternative to cervical cerclage in women with the one who has delivered early or who has lost her pregnancy in the middle of pregnancy and a short cervix (<25 mm) on ultrasound at 20–37 weeks' gestation.

ACOG guideline 2012 recommends daily progesterone supplementation in a woman with history of prior PTB, woman without history of prior PTB but at risk due to short cervix (≤20 mm at ≤24 weeks).

▓ PREVENTION

Emphasis on cervical length (CL) screening has been done based on prior studies. Incidence of birth <35 weeks is 30% in women with CL 20–24 mm, 50% with CL 10–19 mm, and 90% with CL <10 mm. The incidence of birth <35 weeks is only 16% in women with CL >25 mm.[2]

For short cervix <20 mm with no prior PTB, vaginal progesterone/oral/ injectable can be given in any form as follows after identification until 36 weeks: dose of 200 mg suppositories, tablets either oral or vaginally, weekly injections of 17-alpha hydroxyprogesterone caproate. Recent introduction of oral sustained-release seems to be effective, but randomized trials are not done.

▓ TERMINOLOGIES

When preterm labor has been diagnosed?
Diagnosis is when there is a positive evidence of preterm labor.

When preterm labor is established?
If the cervix is dilated more than 4 cm with uterine frequent contraction.

When rupture of membranes occurs preterm?
If there is amniotic fluid leak before 37 weeks of pregnancy.

The following points should be assessed:
If the pregnancy is less than 28 weeks, transfer the women to a tertiary level where the neonatal intensive care unit (NICU) facility to present.

▓ CONTRAINDICATIONS TO STOP LABOR

If there is a harm by continuation of her pregnancy:
- When pregnancy is nonviable
- Cervix is more than 4 cm dilated

- Bleeding from uterus
- Infection is suspected
- Fetal distress
- Rupture of membranes—frank leak of fluid.

INDICATED PRETERM BIRTH[3]

Placental/Obstetric Issues

- Previa alone
- Preterm premature rupture of membranes.

Maternal Issues

- Chronic hypertension (HTN)
- Gestational HTN
- Preeclampsia + severe features.

Fetal Issues

- Intrauterine growth restriction (IUGR) alone
- Multiple pregnancy with IUGR
- Severe oligohydramnios.

DIAGNOSIS

Only 30–60% of women presenting with preterm labor will lead to a PTB. Five main areas of concern that make a difference in survival of infant and they are: (i) transfer to hospital with NICU capabilities, (ii) tocolytics, (iii) antibiotic prophylaxis, (iv) administration of steroids, and (v) magnesium for neuroprotection.[4,5]

Are the membranes ruptured?
The following are observed: pooling of fluid in posterior fornix, ultrasound for amniotic fluid index if unsure.

Is an infection present?
Total count and C-reactive proteins (CRPs) can be done.

Is the patient in labor?
Regular contractions are present or not. If there is contractions, check the cervical dilation.

Diagnosing preterm prelabor rupture of membranes:
A genital examination by a speculum has to be done. If the fluid is pooled in posterior fornix, there is no need to do more tests.

Fetal Fibronectin—24+0 to 33+6 Weeks

Negative predictive value 99% for delivery within 14 days. Positive predictive value 13–30% for delivery in 7–10 days. Can only be done if nothing in vagina in past 24 hours. False positives are seen with amniotic fluid or blood or vaginal infection. Fetal fibronectin (fFN) if available can be offered, which tells that the delivery can occur within 48 hours.

Nonstress Test along with Tocodynamometer for Uterine Contractions Monitoring

Preterm Premature Rupture of Membranes[6]

Preterm premature rupture of membranes prior to 37 weeks and prior to onset of contractions >50% will give birth within 1 week of rupture, 70–80% in 2–5 weeks after intra-amniotic infection in 15–25%, more likely when more preterm.

PPROM—management 24–33+6 weeks: Admission, expectant management unless, nonreassuring fetal status, overt infection, abruption, onset of labor. Single course steroids should be considered. Tocolysis is not recommended in PPROM.

PPROM—other management: Antibiotics, if imminent risk of delivery, magnesium sulfate (MgSO$_4$) for neuroprotection under 32 weeks, delivery by 34 weeks for all PPROM at earlier gestational ages.

Prognosis: Among the preterm labor, 30% resolves spontaneously, 50% of patient hospitalized for preterm labor birth at term, intervention will benefit baby.

Steroids

Single Course 24–34 Weeks at Risk for Delivery in 7 Days

Betamethasone 12 mg intramuscularly (IM) q 24 hours × 2 doses, dexamethasone 6 mg IM q 12 hours × 4 doses. It improves neonatal outcomes. It decreases—mortality, incidence and severity of respiratory distress syndrome (RDS), intraventricular hemorrhage, necrotizing enterocolitis.

Cochrane review 2012: Repeat single course >7 days after initial course.

Rescue steroids: Further reduces RDS without adverse outcomes, should be reserved for imminent delivery. There is no evidence for multiple repeat courses.[7]

Magnesium Sulfate Neuroprophylaxis

Administer when birth is anticipated <32 weeks. MgSO$_4$ reduces severity and risk of cerebral palsy when given for neuroprotection in three meta-analysis. Initially 4 g loading dose then 1 g/hour infusion. Toxicity to be monitored, to be done. This has to be once in 4 hours for pulse, blood pressure (BP), respiration and deep tendon patellar reflexes done. If there is less urine output, reduce $MgSO_4$ dose.

Tocolytics

Used to allow time to give steroids and magnesium, arrange transport if needed.

Contraindications for the same are: previability, IUFD, lethal anomaly, nonreassuring fetal status, chorioamnionitis, preeclampsia with severe features, eclampsia, hemodynamic instability of mother, PPROM, maternal contraindications.

Tocolytic reduce birth within 48 hours but do not improve neonatal outcomes, no evidence for maintenance therapy outside 48–72 hours while inpatient and many risks. Magnesium should no longer be given for tocolysis. When using for neuroprotection, watch interactions with tocolytics.

For tocolysis ideally nifedipine to be started. Atosiban is an alternative. Do not give two drugs together. Dose of nifedipine is 20 mg stat orally and later 10 mg three times a day. Watch for fall of BP.

Indomethacin

Usually used under 32 weeks, after this concern for premature closure of ductus arteriosus. Loading dose 50–100 mg PO, then 25 mg PO q 4–6 hours. This can be used with $MgSO_4$.

NICE Guidelines 2015[8]

Consider nifedipine for tocolysis for women who have intact membranes and are in suspected preterm labor. When nifedipine is contraindicated, atosiban can be used.

Atosiban

The recent drug is atosiban which is an oxytocin receptor antagonist. It is a synthetic peptide.

The action is by a competitive antagonist of oxytocin at uterine oxytocin receptors.

Atosiban Regimen

Preparation of intravenous (IV) infusion of atosiban. Each 0.9 mL vial of atosiban injection contains 6.75 mg. Each 5 mL vial of atosiban solution for infusion contains 37.5 mg (7.5 mg/mL).

Loading dose: Injection Tosiban (37.5 mg/5 mL) 1.5 vials (7.5 mL) in 92.5 mL NS at 12 drops per minute IV infusion for 3 hours (of this 7.5 mL, 0.9 mL may be given over half a minute as an IV bolus starting the 3-hour infusion).

Maintenance dose: Injection Tosiban (37.5 mg/5 mL) 1.5 vials (7.5 mL) in 92.5 mL NS at 4 drops per minute IV infusion for 9 hours. Repeat maintenance dose up to five times—45 hours. Loading + one maintenance dose of 3 + 9 = 11 hours. This regimen is expensive but very effective.

Antibiotic in Preterm Labor

Empirical therapy: There was a reduction in maternal infection (relative risk 0.74, 95% CI 0.64–0.87), but no statistically significant differences in mean gestational age at delivery, frequency of PTB, and neonatal outcomes including mortality. In addition, no differences were noted in a subgroup analysis between the types of antibiotics.

WHO Recommendation on the Prophylactic Antibiotic of Choice in those Pregnant Women with Preterm Prelabor Rupture of Membranes

Erythromycin is recommended as the antibiotic of choice for prophylaxis. Conditional recommendation based on moderate-quality evidence. The use of a combination of amoxicillin and clavulanic acid ("co-amoxiclav") is not recommended.

Analysis of 17 controlled trials which was a meta-analysis of antibiotics in patients at risk of premature birth because of abnormal vaginal flora, previous PTB, or positive fFN, found that there was no association between antibiotic treatment and reduction in PTB irrespective of the criteria used to assess risk, the antimicrobial agent administered, or gestational age at the time of treatment.[9]

A new antibiotic regimen treats and prevents intra-amniotic inflammation/infection in patients with preterm PROM[10,11] (Joon-Ho et al. Published online: 02 December 2015).

Study design—from 1993–2003, ampicillin and/or cephalosporins or a combination was used ("regimen 1"). A new regimen (ceftriaxone, clarithromycin and metronidazole) was used from 2003–2012 ("regimen 2").

Results

1. With the regimens studied there was significance drop in infection with regimen 2, from 68.8 to 52.1% and from 75 to 54.2%, respectively.
2. Intra-amniotic inflammation/infection was eradicated in 33.3% of patients who received regimen 2, but in none who received regimen 1.

Erythromycin is offered by NICE guidelines with PPROM (250 mg) four times a day for a maximum of 10 days or until the woman is in established labor (whichever is sooner).

For women with PPROM who cannot tolerate erythromycin or in whom erythromycin is contraindicated, consider an oral penicillin for a maximum of

10 days or until the woman is in established labor (whichever is sooner) (2015, amended 2019).

RCOG RECOMMENDATION

To diagnosed clinical infection vitals have been monitored along with white blood cell (WBC) and CRP. Fetus should be monitored by cardiotocography (CTG).

Steroids and WBC Count

The WBC count rises following steroid administration and return to normal in 3 days.

C-Reactive Protein

C-reactive protein is the most sensitive marker than total count.[12]

Identifying Infection in Women with PPROM

Assessment of vitals and tests (CRP 1–3 mg/dL) is normal, WBC count, measurement of fetal heart rate using CTG (2015).

When there is a disparity of tests, observation is continued and repeat tests (2015).

DELIVERY MANAGEMENT

Important considerations for preterm delivery, contact NICU, no vacuums <34 weeks, control head extension. Delayed cord clamping is recommended as there is less need for transfusion, less hypotension, less intraventricular hemorrhage, no difference in death. Cord clamping is done after 30 seconds but not longer than 3 minutes. Ideally baby has to be kept below level of the placenta before the cord is clamped.

Fetal monitoring: Fetus should be monitored by CTG or intermittent auscultation.

Mode of birth: Cesarean section if there is no labor pains with severe preterm, malpresentations and if there is severe maternal problems compromising labor.

Cesarean section or normal delivery has to be discussed well.

SUMMARY

- Preterm birth is a serious public health problem. Progesterone is effective in preventing preterm birth. In prior preterm birth, progestogens, cervical length measurements and possible cerclage are the therapeutic alternatives.
- Incidental short cervix: progesterone. Preterm labor: management with intact or not intact membranes, steroids, tocolysis, magnesium for neuroprotection. Management of PPROM is steroids and antibiotics.

■ REFERENCES

1. Norwitz ER, Caughey AB. Progesterone supplementation and the prevention of preterm birth. Rev Obstet Gynecol. 2011;4(2):60-72.
2. Iams JD. Identification of candidates for progesterone: why, who, how, and when? Obstet Gynecol. 2014;123(6):1317-26.
3. American College of Obstetricians and Gynecologists. ACOG committee opinion no. 560: medically indicated late-preterm and early-term deliveries. Obstet Gynecol. 2013;121(4):908-10.
4. Sayres W. Preterm labor. Am Fam Physician. 2010;81:477-84.
5. American College of Obstetricians and Gynecologists; Committee on Practice Bulletins—Obstetrics. ACOG practice bulletin no. 127: management of preterm labor. Obstet Gynecol. 2012;119(6):1308-17.
6. ACOG practice bulletins no. 139: premature rupture of membranes. Obstet Gynecol. 2013;122(4):918-30.
7. McKinlay CJ, Crowther CA, Middleton P, et al. Repeat antenatal glucocorticoids for women at risk of preterm birth: a Cochrane systematic review. Am J Obstet Gynecol. 2012;206(3):187-94.
8. NICE. Preterm labour and birth: NICE guideline [NG25]. (2015). [online] Available from: https://www.nice.org.uk/guidance/ng25 [Last accessed January, 2020].
9. Simcox R, Sin WT, Seed PT, et al. Prophylactic antibiotics for the prevention of preterm birth in women at risk: a meta-analysis. Aust N Z J Obstet Gynaecol. 2007;47:368-77.
10. Lee J, Romero R, Kim SM, et al. A new antibiotic regimen treats and prevents intra-amniotic inflammation/infection in patients with preterm PROM. J Matern Fetal Neonatal Med. 2016;29(17):2727-37.
11. Mercer B. Antibiotics in the management of PPROM and preterm labor. Obstet Gynecol Clin North Am. 2012;39(1):65-76.
12. Royal College of Obstetricians and Gynaecologists (RCOG). Care of women with PROM guideline no 73 (Care of women presenting with suspected preterm prelabour rupture of membranes from 24+0 weeks of gestation (Green-top guideline no. 73). 2019.

2

Induction of Labor

S Shanthakumari, Shraddha Agarwal

"Giving birth should be your greatest achievement and not your greatest fear"
—**Jane Wiedeman**

INTRODUCTION

In the present scenario when there are rising cesarean rates and every woman and doctors want zero complications for mother and baby, we need to revive good techniques for the induction of labor so that the patients who are losing faith on doctors can be given utmost care with lots of patience during induction achieving a normal delivery.

DEFINITION

Induction of labor is defined as the technique of artificially stimulating the uterus to start labor pains. Induction of labor is carried out worldwide for a broad range of maternal and fetal indications, so as to improve pregnancy outcomes.

INDICATIONS

- Prolonged pregnancy (>41 weeks)
- Oligohydramnios
- Gestational hypertension >38 weeks
- Maternal medical condition refractory treatment
- Preterm rupture of membranes
- Prelabor rupture of membranes at term
- Presence of fetal growth restriction
- Alloimmune disease (at or near term)
- Chorioamnionitis
- Uncomplicated twin pregnancy ≥38 weeks
- Previous history of intrauterine demise (IUD)
- Intrauterine fetal demise
- Diabetes mellitus
- Intrauterine growth restriction.

CONTRAINDICATIONS

- Placenta or vasa previa
- Umbilical cord presentation
- Transverse lie or footling breech
- Prior classical or inverted T uterine incision
- Significant prior uterine surgery (e.g. full thickness myomectomy, transfundal uterine surgery)
- Active genital herpes
- Pelvic structural deformities associated with cephalopelvic disproportion
- Invasive cervical carcinoma
- Previous uterine rupture
- Previous pelvic surgeries like vesicovaginal fistula/rectovaginal fistula/pelvic floor repair (third or fourth degree perineal tears repair), trachelorrhaphy.

Induction of labor should not be routinely offered in:
- A diabetic woman with suspected macrosomia
- Convenience of patient or care provider when there is no indication for induction of labor.

PREREQUISITES

- Informed and written consent
- Review of maternal history and profile
- Evaluation for indications and rule out any contraindications
- Reliable estimation of gestational age (by earlier scans), presentation, and fetal weight
- Maternal pulse, blood pressure, temperature, respiratory rate, and findings on abdominal palpation must be recorded
- Evaluation of baseline fetal heart rate pattern by auscultation/electronic fetal monitoring [Cardiotocography (CTG)]
- Maternal pelvis assessment and clinical evaluation for possible cephalopelvic or fetopelvic disproportion.

TIMING OF INDUCTION

- According to the Cochrane review 2012, it is recommended to induce women with uncomplicated pregnancies at or beyond 41 weeks.
- In case of term prelabor rupture of membranes, incidence of chorio-amnionitis and endometritis and neonatal sepsis is reduced if labor is induced.
- In cases of previous cesarean section, rates of repeat cesarean section are reduced but risk of neonatal complications increases.

- In cases of hypertensive disorders, more than 34 weeks of gestation, elective induction is associated with lower rate of complications.
- In cases of breech presentation, rate of cesarean section is high in induction group.
- In cases of uncomplicated twin gestation, there is no harm in induction beyond 37 weeks of pregnancy.

CERVICAL RIPENING

A ripened cervix is a boon for any obstetrician and her patient for inducing labor, so assessment of cervix is the very next step after confirming the indication for induction of labor.

Assessment of cervical status using Modified Bishop scoring system **(Table 1)** to predict the likelihood of success and select appropriate method of induction of labor.

Assessment of Bishop's Score

Total score = 13
Favorable score = 6–13
Unfavorable score = 0–5
A score of <5 suggests further ripening is needed, while a score of 9 or greater suggests that ripening is complete.
One point is added to the total score for:
- Existence of preeclampsia
- Each previous vaginal delivery

One point is subtracted from the total score for:
- Postdated/post-term pregnancy
- Nulliparity (no previous vaginal deliveries)
- *PPROM*: Preterm premature rupture of membranes.

Cervix	Score			
	0	*1*	*2*	*3*
Cervical dilatation	0	1–2	3–4	<1
Cervical length (cm)	>4	2–4	1–2	<1
Station of presenting part (cm in relation to ischial spine)	-3 or above	-2	-1, 0	+1, +2
Consistency		Firm	Medium	Soft
Position		Posterior	Midposition	anterior

TABLE 1: Modified Bishop Score.

■ METHODS OF CERVICAL RIPENING AND INDUCTION OF LABOR IN UNFAVORABLE CERVIX

Cervical ripening refers to the softening of cervix that typically begins prior to the onset of labor contractions and is necessary for cervical dilatation and the passage of the fetus. It is the result of realignment of collagen, degradation of collagen cross-linking due to proteolytic enzymes, and uterine contractions. There is an increase in prostaglandin E2 (PGE2) in the cervix, which leads to dilatation of small vessels in the cervix, increase in collagen degradation, increase in hyaluronic acid, and many more events like increase in PGF2-alpha, which leads to increase in glycosaminoglycans.

Induction of Cervical Ripening

Cervical ripening allows uterine contractions to effectively dilate the cervix. The amount of uterine pressure required to dilate a ripe cervix is thought to be approximately 1,600 mm Hg as compared to 10,000 mm Hg required for an unripe cervix.

There are various methods:

Prostaglandins

- *Prostaglandin E2*: Two forms are available commercially in our country.
  - Cerviprime, which comes in the form of gel and is placed inside the cervix but not above the internal os. The application (3 g gel/0.5 mg dinoprostone) can be repeated in 6 h, not to exceed three doses in 24 h.
  - Propess (Dinoprostone vaginal pessary), which comes in the form of mesh and contains dinoprostone 10 mg is placed in the posterior fornix of vagina which allows controlled release of dinoprostone over 24 h, after which it is removed. Controlled release of dinoprostone minimizes the risk of hyperstimulation in comparison to intracervical or intravaginal gels as the pessary can easily be removed when labor starts or at the onset of any adverse event. Single dose is needed and easy to insert in OPD itself.

  Combination of oxytocin and PGE2 results in increased chances of vaginal deliveries within 24 h.
- *Prostaglandin E1 (Misoprostol)* is a synthetic prostaglandin, 25 µg can be crushed and placed on the cervix. It is effective in cervical ripening and labor, and the application can be repeated every 4 hours. The major risk of the use of misoprostol is hyperstimulation soothe woman and fetus must be monitored for contractions, fetal well-being, and changes in cervical Bishop score. It should not be used in cases of previous cesarean section or major uterine surgery.

  Combination of oxytocin induction preceded by a misoprostol induction is safe and shortens induction-to-delivery time.

Low Dose Oxytocin Infusion

Dose of oxytocin from 1 to 4 mU/min is comparable to intravaginal misoprostol used for cervical priming.

Balloon Catheter

A 30–50 mL Foley's catheter filled with saline is effective in inducing cervical ripening and dilatation. The balloon is placed in the uterus, which causes direct stress in the lower uterine segment and cervix and results in the release of local prostaglandins. The PROBAAT trial compared the effectiveness and safety of induction of labor using a Foley's catheter with induction using vaginal prostaglandin E2 gel and found that in women with unfavorable cervix at term, results were similar.

Membrane Stripping

Manual separation of the amniotic membranes from cervix is thought to induce cervical ripening and the onset of labor. Authors of a Cochrane database review concluded that this practice provides no clinically important benefits.
Other methods:
- Hygroscopic dilators (laminaria tents), mifepristone, nitric oxide donors, relaxin, hyaluronidase or breast nipple stimulation are presently not recommended for induction of labor in view of the availability of low quality evidence for their use.

■ INDUCTION OF LABOR WITH A FAVORABLE CERVIX

Nonpharmacological Methods

- Mechanical dilators like 18F Foley's catheter is used widely for induction of labor. The Foley's catheter is inserted into cervical os and balloon is inflated with saline, then it is pulled and traction is given to facilitate the stretching of internal os. The Foley's catheter is left in situ for 12–24 h. A Cochrane review of 71 studies showed that the use of mechanical dilators had similar efficacy of vaginal delivery with similar cesarean section rates and minimal uterine hyperstimulation as compared to prostaglandins.
- Hygroscopic dilators like laminaria tents derived from seaweed are not used nowadays.
- Amniotomy:
  - A simple and effective method when the membranes are accessible and the cervix is favorable. It creates a commitment to delivery.[1]
  - Flow of amniotic fluid should be controlled with vaginal fingers. The liquor should be drained slowly because sudden decompression of uterus can lead to placenta abruption.

- Care should be taken when amniotomy is done in unengaged presentation because there is a risk of cord prolapse. The vaginal fingers should not be removed until presenting part rests against the cervix.
- Amount and color (meconium or blood stained) of the liquor is observed.
- Monitoring of fetal heart should be done during and after the procedure.
- Oxytocin should be commenced immediately after amniotomy or after 2 hours depending on the intensity of uterine contractions.

There is not enough evidence as per Cochrane review 2000 to suggest that amniotomy alone is an efficacious method to induce labor.[2]

- *Membrane sweeping and stretching*: It involves introducing a finger under aseptic conditions in cervix beyond internal os and sweeping through the uterus circumferentially which results in release of PGF2 alpha and initiation of uterine contractions.[3] A Cochrane review of 22 studies of 2,797 women showed that membrane stripping at term reduced the rate of formal induction of labor at 41 weeks. There were no maternal side effects of the procedure. However, it is not recommended method for Rh incompatible pregnancy for fear of Rh isoimmunization.
- *Nipple stimulation*: Releases oxytocin and helps in the stimulation of labor.

Pharmacological Methods of Induction of Labor[4-7]

- *Prostaglandins*: They have the dual advantage of increasing uterine smooth muscle contractility and cervical ripening.[8]
    - *Prostaglandin E2 or dinoprostone*: It initiates uterine contraction and is available as 0.5 mg gel and 10 mg vaginal pessary.[9] Comparable outcomes are found between the Foley's and prostaglandin E2 for mean induction time and cesarean section rate; when compared with *misoprostol* and prostaglandin E2 takes longer time to achieve active phase, a longer induction time, and higher risk for cesarean section. Oxytocin can be started 30 min after the removal of a dinoprostone insert and 6 h after gel. Fetal heart and uterine activity should be monitored after 30 min to 2 h after insertion.
        - Side effects include transient fall in blood pressure, nausea and vomiting, and fever.
        - Caution in needed in women with glaucoma, severe hepatic and renal function and asthma.
    - *Prostaglandin E1 (misoprostol)*: Evidence shows that misoprostol is safe and effective agent for labor induction with intact membranes and on an inpatient basis. It is more effective than PGE2 to achieve vaginal delivery and results in less epidural use but more uterine hyperstimulation. Oral and vaginal routes have a similar reduction in cesarean section rates. The lower vaginal dose 25 μg tends to need more oxytocin stimulation

than the high vaginal dose (>50 μg). Electronic fetal monitoring should be performed for 30 min after administration of misoprostol and for 60 min after any tachysystole. Network meta-analysis 2016 found that the misoprostol might be the best prostaglandin for labor induction. It should not be used in the setting vaginal birth after cesarean section due to increased risk of uterine rupture. Oxytocin should be started after 4 hours of last dose of misoprostol.

- *Oxytocin*
  - Intravenous oxytocin is the most commonly used method of induction for women with a favorable cervix (Modified Bishop Score >6).
  - Oxytocin can be used alone, in combination with amniotomy, or following cervical ripening. It can be used for induction as well as augmentation of labor.
  - It should be used with caution in women with previous cesarean delivery and grand multiparous women because of the risk of uterine rupture.
  - Oxytocin should be administered intravenously as an infusion to allow continuous, precise control of the dose administered.
  - The low-dose regimen begins with 1–2 mU/min, increased incrementally by 1–2 mU at every 30 min intervals.
  - The high-dose regimen starts with 4–6 mU/min with dose increments of 4–6 mU/min every 15–30 min.
  - High dose protocols reduce the induction delivery interval and are associated with higher rates of tachysystole than low dose protocols. Maternal and fetal complication rates are similar with both protocols.
  - The oxytocin infusion can be increased until labor progress is normal or uterine activity reaches 200–250 Montevideo units (i.e., good regular uterine contractions, each lasting for 40–45 seconds duration and minimum of three contractions in 10 minutes.
  - Monitoring for infusion rate of oxytocin and uterine contractions and fetal heart rate by continuous cardiotocography is preferable method.
  - Blood pressure and pulse should be assessed every hour. Intake and output should be assessed every 4 hours. The frequency, intensity, and duration of uterine contractions should be assessed every 30 minutes and with each incremental increase in oxytocin.
  - Cervical status should be assessed prior to administration of oxytocin and repeated after at least 4 hours of moderate contractions.
  - A vaginal examination may also be repeated in situation of a nonreassuring fetal heart pattern to rule out the presence of meconium, abruption or a cord accident.
  - Close watch is kept for clinical features of maternal hyponatremia, uterine hyperstimulation, and uterine rupture.

- Oxytocin is administered as dilute solution by intravenous route. Isotonic solutions such as ringer lactate or normal saline are preferred over dextrose solution for fluid selection to minimize the risk of electrolyte imbalance (e.g. hyponatremia) and volume overload.
- 2 mL of oxytocin (two ampoules) is taken in a 10 mL syringe and diluted with 8 mL of normal saline. It makes 10 mL of saline solution having 10 units of oxytocin. One mL of this saline solution contains one unit of oxytocin. To make a bottle of two units of oxytocin infusion, 2 mL of this solution is added in 500 mL of Ringer lactate.[10,11]

MONITORING DURING INDUCTION OF LABOR

- Before induction of labor, a nonstress test is recommended.
- Intermittent maternal and fetal (fetal heart rate) monitoring should be done every hour initially.
- Continuous electronic/more frequent intermittent fetal heart rate monitoring should be started in active labor.
- Progress of labor is monitored using partogram.
- Close watch is kept for temperature, pulse rate, blood pressure, fetal heart pattern, vaginal bleeding, uterine hyperstimulation, uterine rupture, and scar dehiscence in women with previous cesarean delivery.

PAIN RELIEF AFTER INDUCTION

- Women should be provided pain relief appropriate for them after counseling. This can range from simple analgesics to epidural analgesia.
- Women should be encouraged to use breathing and relaxation techniques in labor.
- There is no need to wait for labor analgesia arbitrarily till the cervical dilation has reached 4–5 cm.
- If regional analgesia is planned, the woman should be informed about the risks and benefits and the implications for her in labor.

COMPLICATIONS

- *Uterine hyperstimulation*:
  - First step is to discontinue oxytocin infusion or withdraw dinoprostone vaginal pessary.
  - Tocolytics preferably betamimetics are recommended for women with uterine hyperstimulation during induction of labor. Contraindications of betamimetics especially cardiac disease should be kept in mind.
  - If associated with abnormal fetal heart pattern, decision for cesarean section is taken.

- *Uterine rupture*:
  - Rupture can occur in both scarred and unscarred uterus and is associated with multiparity, malpresentation, unsupervised or aggressive use of uterotonics.
  - A close watch is kept on maternal signs and monitoring is done for fetal heart rate abnormality.
  - In suspected case of uterine rupture or scar dehiscence, delivery is by emergency cesarean section.
- *Uterine atony*:
  - Postpartum atony and hemorrhage are more common in women undergoing induction or augmentation.
  - Increased risk of cesarean section
  - Chorioamnionitis.

FAILED INDUCTION

It means that the latent phase has continued for an extended length of time and after clinical assessment, it is unlikely that active phase will be reached to achieve a successful vaginal delivery.[12]

Failed induction of labor must be differentiated from failure of progress of labor (prolonged active phase, prolonged second stage, nonreassuring fetal status). Latent phase of labor of cervical ripening is excluded from diagnosing failed induction.

The definition in case of prostaglandins is "failure to induce progressive labor after one cycle of treatment" consisting of the insertion of two vaginal PGE2 tablets (3 mg) or gel (1–2 mg) at 6 h interval or one PGE2 controlled released pessary (10 mg) over 24 h.

- Maternal and fetal well-being should be reassessed.
- Subsequent management options are: Another attempt to induce labor with a different method can be considered after discussion with the patient but it depends on the nature and urgency of the clinical situation (indication of the induction of labor) cesarean delivery.

CONCLUSION

Induction of labor should only be offered when there is clear medical indication and benefits for the mother and baby outweigh its potential harms, and this requires careful consideration of the clinical evidence in discussion with the woman.

"You are a birth servant. Do good without show or fuss. If you must take the lead, lead so that the mother is helped, yet still free and incharge. When the baby is born, they will rightly say; we did it ourselves!." TaoTe Ching

■ REFERENCES

1. Mundle S, Bracken H, Khedikar V, Mulik J, Faragher B, Easterling T, et al. Foley catheterization versus oral misoprostol for induction of labour in hypertensive women in India (INFORM); Lancet. 2017;390;669-80.
2. Bricker L, Luckas M. Amniotomy alone for induction of labour. Cochrane Database Syst Rev. 2000;4:CD 002862.
3. Boulvain M, Stan CM, Irion O. Membrane sweeping for induction of labour. Cochrane Database Syst. Rev 2005:(1);CD 000451.
4. Alfirevic Z, Kelly AJ, Dowswell T. Intravenous oxytocin alone for cervical ripening and induction of labor. Cochrane Database Syst Rev. 2009;(4): CD003246.
5. American College of Obstetricians and Gynecologists Committee on obstetric practice. ACOG committee opinion No 342. Induction of labor for vaginal birth after cesarean delivery. Obstet Gynecol. 2006;108(2):465-8.
6. Christensen FC, Tehranifar M, Gonzalez JL, Qualls CR, Rappaport VJ, Rayburn WF. Randomized trial of concurrent oxytocin with a sustained release dinoprostone vaginal insert for labor induction at term. Am J Obstet Gynecol. 2002;186(1);61-5.
7. Laughon SK, Zhang J, Troendle J, Sun L, Redduy UM. Using a simplified bishop score to predict vaginal delivery. Obstet Gynaecol. 2011;117(4):805-11.
8. Alfirevic Z, Keeney E, Dowswell T, Welton NJ, Medley N, Dias S, et al. Methods to induce labour: a systematic review. Network meta-analysis and cost effectiveness analysis. BJOG. 2016;123:1462-70.
9. Dallenbach P, Boulvain M, Viardot C, Irion O. Oral misoprostol or vaginal dinoprostone for labour induction: a randomized controlled trial. Am J Obstet Gyanecol. 2003;188:162-7.
10. Budden A, Chen LJ, Henry A. High dose versus low dose oxytocin infusion regimens for induction of labour at term. Cochrane Database Syst Rev. 2014;(10):CD009701.
11. Freeman RK, Nageotte M, A protocol for use of oxytocin. Am J Obstet Gynecol. 2007;197(5):445.
12. Rouse DJ, Owen J, Houth JC. Criteria for failed labour induction. Prospective evaluation of a standardized protocol. Obstet Gyanecol. 2000;96(5 Pt 1):671.

Consent Form

I (Name of the patient) wife of Sh. (Name of the husband) ID No: ....
.... have read the above document and have
understood the need for the proposed procedure. The indication, possible
complications and need for further procedure in case of failure of the induction
of labor have been explained to us by our doctor (Name of the doctor). I have
been given the opportunity to ask questions and clarify my doubts. I hearty
give my full consent to undergo the procedure. I understand the risk involved.
Procedure (specify the method of induction of labor):

Indication:

Time and date:

Place:

Name and signature of the patient   Name and signature of the attendant

Name and signature of the doctor   Name and signature of the witness

Check List

Method used for the patient: ....

Name of patient: .... w/o: ....

ID No. ....; Date: ....; Time: ....

- Age (Date of birth): .... years; Gravida and parity: ....
- LMP (last menstrual period): ....
- Expected date of delivery: ....
- Corrected expected date of delivery: ....
- Gestational age by LMP: ....
- Gestational age by first ultrasound (done before 20 weeks of gestation): ...
  ....
- History of any allergies, medical condition, special need: Yes/No
- High risk review: Yes/No
- Indication for induction reviewed: Yes/No
- Planned method of induction: Yes/ No
- Consent form signed by the patient and her attendant: Yes/No
- Fetal heart rate assessment: Yes/No
- Pre-induction modified Bishop's score:

Total score of patient: Favorable score and unfavorable score

Signature of doctor: Date and time:

Name of doctor:

3

Current Practice of Cesarean Section

Rajkumar H Shah, Mohan A Gadam ■

■ OVERVIEW

The term "cesarean" may refer to the patients being cut open, because the Latin verb "caedare" means to cut. *"Cesarean operation"* was the preferred term before 1598 publication of Guillimeau, who later introduced the term *"cesarean section (CS)".*

The term cesarean delivery originally was believed to have been derived from the birth of Julius Caesar; however it is unlikely that his mother Aurelia would have survived the operation. During those times, CS was reserved for a dead or a dying mother. Roman law under Numa Pompilius, the first (Lex Regia), and then renamed after Caesar (Lex Cesarea), specified surgical removal of the fetus before the death of a diseased pregnant woman.

The rapid increase in cesarean birth rates from 1996 to 2014 without clear evidence of concomitant decreases in maternal or neonatal morbidity or mortality raises significant concern that cesarean delivery is overused.

With minor variations, surgical performance of cesarean delivery is comparable worldwide. Most steps are founded on evidence-based data, and these have been reviewed by Dahlke (2013) and Hofmeyr (2009) and their associates.

This being a reference book, the surgical steps are not discussed in detail. Efforts have been made to highlight each and every step from the point of view of evidence-based approach.

■ CHANGING TRENDS IN INDICATIONS FOR CESAREAN SECTION

- *Difficult labor or dystocia*: In the developed world, dystocia or poor progress in labor contributes at least a third of the overall CS rate. Dystocia is classified as a protraction disorder or as an arrest disorder. These can be primary or secondary disorders. When a diagnosis of dystocia in labor is made, the indication should be detailed according to the previous classification that is, primary or secondary disorder, arrest or protraction disorder, or a combination of the above.
- *Fetal distress*: Access to electronic fetal monitoring (EFM) is held responsible for rising CS rates for fetal distress.

- *Previous CS*: Maternal preference may play a part as CS is regarded as a safe and convenient procedure and for the clinician, is less likely to give rise to complications such as dehiscence and possible subsequent litigation.
- *Premature* (Breech, cephalic presentation) when associated with other clinical circumstances such as placental abruption or severe pre-eclampsia, may be responsible for resorting to CS.
- *Multiple pregnancy*: Incidence is on the rise due to assisted conception and increasing maternal age. Besides themselves being indication for CS, chorionicity, other maternal and fetal indications, gestation, and final presentation of both twins at delivery are considered.
- *Cord around the neck*: The enormous anxieties mothers go through when their fetuses have locked pattern of nuchal cords continue to challenge obstetricians. From the perspective of neonatologists, who see evidence of tight nuchals as in tCAN syndrome (Tight Cord Around the Neck Syndrome) and pathologists who witness during autopsy, tight nuchal cord as a cause of stillbirth, nuchal cords *do not seem to be benign*. If the rampant increase in CS for this cause is to be limited, *diagnosing nuchal cords by judicious use of ultrasound with color Doppler, middle cerebral artery (MCA), and umbilical artery (UA) resistance index ratios, amniotic erythropoietin (EPO) levels, and possibly the use of manual abdomen compression or vibroacoustic stimulation tests* will hold a key role.[1]
- *Fetal conditions*:
  - *Macrosomia*: It has been suggested that a policy of prophylactic CS in babies with an estimated weight of 4–4.5 kg would require more than 1,000 cesarean deliveries to avoid a single case of brachial nerve damage.[2] This is true for American population. How it applies to others, has to be studied.
  - *Transverse lie*: A judicious resort to external cephalic version either antenatally or intrapartum prior to a CS for abnormal presentation, using tocolysis and ultrasound, has been shown to reduce CS rates by 50%.[3]
  - *Fetal anomalies*: The decision about mode of delivery is dictated by the need for highly skilled pediatric assistance at the time of birth and the timing of reconstructive surgery in the newborn period.
- *Maternal request*: When a woman requests a CS when there is no other indication, it is pertinent to discuss the overall risks and benefits of CS compared with vaginal delivery and record that this discussion has taken place. Include a discussion with another obstetrician and anesthetist, to explore the reasons for the request and provide the woman with accurate information. She may be referred to an expert, providing perinatal mental health support to address her anxiety in a supportive manner. In spite of these measures, if the woman still does not accept vaginal birth, offer a planned CS or refer the patient to another obstetrician who will carry out the CS.[4]

- *Mother-to-child transmission (MTCT) of maternal infections*:
  - *HIV*: CS should not be offered on the grounds of HIV status to prevent MTCT, as there is insufficient evidence that it prevents MTCT. Only those women with HIV who are *not* on any antiretroviral therapy or on any ART and have viral load of about 400 copies/mL or more may benefit from CS in preventing MTCT.
  - *Hepatitis B, C virus*: Women with hepatitis B or C should not be offered a planned CS as it does not reduce the MTCT (2004). However, women who are coinfected with hepatitis C virus and HIV should be offered planned CS because it reduces MTCT of both (2004).

■ TECHNIQUE OF PERFORMING CESAREAN SECTION

General Principles

- Counseling the patient is a good clinical practice and essential in risk management. Seek for appropriate assistance and be in readiness to call for help when in difficulty.
- It is advisable to revise patient's history especially with respect to previous surgery, if any. Highlight relevant points and risk factors in the history. It is important to note the location of the placenta.
- Individualize technique depending on following factors: Gestational age, fetal presentation and position, size and number of fetuses, maternal health, and degree of urgency.
- Anticipation and proper planning are key factors to avoid complications. A point in example is if a CS is being done in a woman who has prolonged rupture of membranes with oligoamnios, delivery of the fetus may pose a problem due to a tight hugging uterus. If the anesthetist is forewarned of the need for uterine relaxation, then it will be kept ready before the incision is made!

Avoiding Injuries to the Operating Team

Contact with sharp objects has to be minimized. Use of scissors vis-à-vis scalpel for fascia, peritoneum, and myometrium is safer. Sharp instruments should be transferred in basin or tray. Use retractors as against fingers, or hand for tissue retraction.

Needle stick injuries can be avoided:

- By mounting needle on holder after use
- By using forceps to reposition needle
- By using metal thimble when counter pressure is required
- Cut-off the needle from suture material and handover to scrub-nurse before tying the knot
- Using double gloves, reduces the puncture of inner glove by a factor of six.[5]

Position of Patient

Supine position leads to hypotension, hypoperfusion of placenta, and decreases fetal oxygenation. A standard practice is to give a 10–15º lateral tilt. In this position, fewer low Apgar scores and better cord pH measurements were seen.[6] A left lateral tilt is better than right lateral tilt. Use of manual displacers can be used to achieve a left lateral tilt.[7]

Skin Preparation

Shaving is not mandatory and infection rates are lowest, if shaving is done just prior to the surgery. Depilatory agents are better than using razor.[8] Povidone-iodine with tincture chlorhexidine gluconate is usually recommended. Alcohol and hexachlorophene are used only if patient is hypersensitive to above agents. If 10% alcohol is used, diathermy should be used only on full evaporation. For rapid skin preparation, iodophor impregnated film can be used. Use of antibiotics for pelvic irrigation was associated with less incidence of endometritis.[9]

Skin Incision

A CS can be performed by various incisions mentioned below:
- Midline subumbilical vertical **(Table 1)**
- Low transverse curvilinear incision (Pfannenstiel) **(Table 2)**
- Maylard's incision
- Frank's Straight transverse incision
- Joel-Cohen's incision.

TABLE 1: Midline subumbilical vertical incision.

Advantages	Indications
Less vascular	Massive hemorrhage
Rapid entry	Exploration of upper abdomen
Good exposure to abdomen and pelvis	Perimortem CS
	Patients on anticoagulant
	Refusing blood transfusions

TABLE 2: Pfannenstiel incision.

Advantages	Disadvantages
Excellent cosmetic results	Extensive dissection
Early ambulation	Injuries to ilioinguinal and iliohypogastric nerves
Low incidence of wound disruption, dehiscence, and hernia	Limits view of upper abdomen
	Increased blood loss and hematoma rates

Joel-Cohen's Incision (1954)

This is a straight transverse incision, slightly higher than Pfannenstiel.

The subcutaneous tissue is not divided by sharp cutting but by blunt dissection. The anterior rectus sheath is incised in the midline for 3 cm and the muscles are not separated from the sheath. The peritoneum is bluntly opened transversely and also widened transversely. The advantages are there is less fever, pain, and analgesic requirements; less blood loss; and shorter duration of surgery and hospital stay.[10]

Modified Joel-Cohen incision (Wallin and Fall): The incision is made 3 cm above pubic symphysis. The peritoneum is opened bluntly. There is no closure of parietal and visceral peritoneum. In comparison to the Pfannenstiel incision, the Joel-Cohen incision is associated with less blood loss, shorter operating time, reduced time to oral intake, less risk of fever, shorter duration of postoperative pain, lower analgesic requirements, and shorter time from skin incision to birth of the baby.[11,12]

Maylard Incision

It involves cutting rectus muscles transversely, ligating inferior epigastric artery, and proceeding further. It gives good pelvic access and is a safe option when risk factors, viz. macrosomic baby or twins needing maximal exposure for nontraumatic delivery are being considered. However, there is greater discomfort postoperatively.[13] In fact, the transection of the rectus muscles is associated with increased blood loss.[14]

Length of Skin Incision

Broadly speaking, the incision should be adequate, meaning thereby, it should be as long as an Allis clamp laid on the skin (6" or 15 cm). A uterine incision delivery interval was shorter in the group that passed the "Allis test" versus the group that failed the test (58.4 s vs. 95.7 s, $p = 0.002$).[15] Blunt dissection tends to be associated with reduced blood loss.[16]

Uterine Incision

Either a transverse (Munro Kerr) or a vertical (Kronig *or* DeLee) incision may be made on the uterus. The choice of incision is based on several factors—fetal presentation, gestational age, placental location, and presence of a well-developed lower uterine segment.

The Lower Segment Transverse Uterine Incision (Munro Kerr 1926)

The transverse uterine incision is made in the center 2–3 cm till membranes are exposed. The deeper fibers of myometrium should be opened bluntly by fingers/butt of scalpel to avoid injury to fetus.

If sharp dissection is required, use thick bandage scissors to cut the thick lower segment. In difficult situations, if extension of incision is required, a J-shaped extension into upper segment is better than an inverted T. The latter forms weaker scars due to poor healing. Both are frequently associated with intraoperative complications and prolonged hospital stay.[17]

The Lower Segment Vertical Uterine Incision

A vertical incision may be chosen if the lower segment is not well developed, if an anterior placenta previa is present or if the fetus is in a transverse lie or in a preterm nonvertex presentation. It is initiated with a scalpel in the inferior portion of the lower uterine segment. Care is taken to avoid injury to the underlying fetus and the incision is carried into the uterus until the cavity is entered. The incision is extended superiorly with sharp dissection. If the incision is confined to the lower uterine segment, patients can be counseled for a trial of labor and vaginal delivery in subsequent pregnancies. The risk of uterine rupture is similar to that associated with a transverse incision, with most recent reports finding a risk for uterine rupture of less than 1.5%.[18]

A vertical incision may also be considered when a hysterectomy may be planned in the setting of a placenta accreta or when the patient has a coexisting cervical cancer for which a hysterectomy would be an appropriate treatment. This incision is associated with a greater degree of blood loss and a longer operating time than a low transverse incision, but poses less risk of injury to the uterine vessels.

■ DELIVERY OF FETUS

Some important aspects of delivery are:
- The incision to delivery time (especially in antenatally compromised fetuses)
- Delivery of an impacted fetal head.

An incision-delivery interval of more than 3 minutes in general anesthesia or spinal anesthesia is associated with low Apgar scores and neonatal acidosis.[19,20] However, Vatashsky and coworkers and Anderson and coworkers concluded that the incision-delivery interval did not significantly affect the outcome.

Fetuses should always be delivered in occipitoanterior position.

In a high floating head, a Wrigley's forceps or the use of one blade as Vectis or a Ventouse may be used. This however increases the incision-delivery interval with its known problems.[21] Difficulties should be anticipated, discussed with patient and anesthetist, and certain provisions, viz. instruments like forceps, vacuum should be made available on the instrument trolley before the patient is anesthetized. When in difficulty, the general principle is to request the anesthetist for uterine relaxation. A glyceryl-trinitrate drip or the use of halothane/isoflurane/sevoflurane by inhalational mask may be helpful.

During a CS for a face/brow presentation, it is imperative to flex the fetal head and deliver. For a breech delivery at CS, maneuvers to deliver are the same as vaginal delivery, by delivering feet, pelvis, shoulder, and then the after coming head. Difficult breech deliveries in emergency CS or after rupture of membranes should be anticipated. The assistant should give fundal pressure while the surgeon delivers the fetus by jaw flexion, shoulder traction or by planned forceps delivery of the after coming head.

For a transverse lie, an external cephalic version should be tried before incision. If unsuccessful, consider internal podalic version with breech extraction. A deeply engaged head in the late second stage of labor may pose a difficulty in delivering the baby. Delivery can be achieved by the fetal head being pushed by an assistant or by a Patwardhan maneuver with breech extraction.

Certain injuries to the fetus at uterine incision, viz. scalp wounds are *not considered expected complications*. Similarly, difficult extraction may cause fracture of long bones of the fetus or tendon lacerations. In the eventuality of such occurrences, it is important to inform the patient, the circumstances leading to such mishaps and the corrective measures that have been carried out and a clear documentation to that effect should be done.

PLACENTAL EXTRACTION

Removal of placenta by spontaneous expulsion with gentle traction is shown to be associated with less blood loss and a lower rate of endometritis than manual extraction as shown by randomized controlled trials (RCTs).[22,23]

Spontaneous delivery, along with some cord traction, may reduce the risk of operative blood loss and infection (Anorlu, 2008; Baksu, 2005). Fundal massage may begin as soon as the fetus is delivered to hasten placental separation and delivery. Many surgeons often prefer manual removal of placenta, which is shown to be of no benefit. Therefore, spontaneous expulsion with gentle cord traction and uterine massage should always be the method of delivery of placenta.

A common practice of changing gloves has been studied and intraoperative glove change has not shown to decrease the risk of endometritis.

EXTERIORIZATION OF THE UTERUS

After the placental delivery, the uterus is lifted through the incision onto the draped abdominal wall, and the fundus is covered with a moistened laparotomy sponge. Although some clinicians prefer to avoid such uterine exteriorization, it often has benefits that outweigh its disadvantages.

Uterine repair may be greatly facilitated by exteriorization. It can facilitate better visualization of the extent of the uterine incision to be repaired and can provide a better view of the adnexa. For example, the relaxed, atonic uterus can be recognized quickly, and massage applied. The incision and bleeding points are more easily visualized and repaired, especially if there have been extensions. As adnexal exposure is superior, tubal sterilization is easier.

There is no significant increased risk for blood loss, infection, hypotension or nausea and vomiting that has been reported with exteriorization compared with intra-abdominal repair as shown by a meta-analysis of 11 trials.[24]

This issue is however controversial and the decision regarding uterine exteriorization can hence be based on a surgeon's preference.

Bleeding along the incision line is temporarily controlled with the help of ring forceps. The uterus is then manually curetted with a moistened sponge to remove remaining placental fragments and the membranes. Dilatation of the cervix is not associated with any additional benefit.[25,26]

It does not improve infection rates from potential hematometra and is not recommended (Güngördük, 2009; Liabsuetrakul, 2011).

■ SUTURING OF UTERINE INCISION

The first layer of the uterine incision is best closed with continuous noninterlocking stitch with 1-0 or 0-0 delayed absorbable suture, going well beyond the edges on either side. Enough tension is applied to just obliterate the vessels without strangulating the tissue. It is important to carefully select the site of each stitch and to avoid withdrawing the needle once it penetrates the myometrium. This minimizes perforation of unligated vessels and subsequent bleeding. The running locked or unlocked suture is continued just beyond the opposite incision angle. This technique is associated with less operative time and reduced blood loss compared to interrupted suturing.[27]

Locking of the primary layer may not be necessary if the incision is hemostatic before the closure. Locking with use of excessive force may lead to fibrosis causing weakness of cesarean scar and hence should be avoided. Full thickness repair including the endometrial layer is associated with improved healing as evidenced by ultrasound 6 weeks after cesarean delivery.[28] Some concerns have been expressed by clinicians that sutures through the decidua may lead to endometriosis or adenomyosis in the hysterotomy scar, but this is rare.

Single Layer or Double Layer Closure—The Debate Continues!

The single layer closure is associated with statically significant but clinically small reduction in mean blood loss, duration of operative procedure, and presence of postoperative pain compared with double-layer closure.[29]

Controversy surrounds the fact, an increased risk for subsequent uterine rupture or placenta accreta accompanies the single layer closure technique. The policy to adopt would be single layer closure if perfect hemostasis is achieved and the patient is not interested in future childbearing. Otherwise a double-layered closure is resorted to.

However, RCTs that have assessed single layer versus double-layered closure have reported mostly short-term outcomes with insufficient evidence to assess long-term outcomes, particularly in relation to uterine rupture with a trial of labor after cesarean (TOLAC) [vaginal birth after cesarean (VBAC)] in the future pregnancy.[25]

Closure of Classical Incision

A vertical uterine incision (classical) generally requires at least a double-layered closure and more often a triple-layered closure technique with a baseball stich used on the serosa.

After confirming hemostasis, the uterus is returned to the peritoneal cavity. Individual bleeding points are cauterized or ligated. The adnexa are inspected, and the abdominal closure is performed after an instrument count and the mop count. Intra-abdominal irrigation does not reduce intrapartum or postpartum morbidity.

■ PREVENTION OF ADHESIONS

Adhesions following cesarean delivery commonly form within the vesicouterine space or between the anterior abdominal wall and uterus. With each successive pregnancy, the percentage of affected women and adhesion severity increases (Morales, 2007; Tulandi, 2009). Adhesions can significantly lengthen incision-to-delivery times and total operative time (Rossouw, 2013; Sikirica, 2012).

Although occurring infrequently, rates of cystotomy and bowel injury are also increased (Rahman, 2009; Silver, 2006). Intuitively, scarring can be reduced by handling tissues delicately, achieving hemostasis, and minimizing tissue ischemia, infection, and foreign body reaction. Using basic principles of surgery: Perfect and meticulous hemostasis, thorough asepsis, and anatomical closure are the hallmarks of any surgical technique and thus should always be resorted to.

Data are conflicting reports regarding closure of the bladder flap (visceral peritoneum) or of the abdominal cavity (parietal peritoneum) and its effect on subsequent adhesions. Some note benefit from closure of one, but not the other, or neither (CAESAR study collaborative group, 2010; Cheong, 2009; Kapustian, 2012; Lyell, 2005, 2012). Benefit from placement of an adhesion barrier at the repaired hysterotomy site is limited to only two nonrandomized studies (Chapa, 2011; Fushiki, 2005).

Currently, there is an ongoing multicenter randomized trial to evaluate use of the barrier Seprafilm at the time of cesarean delivery (National Institutes of Health, 2012).

Best efforts must always be made to prevent formation of adhesions as it will have substantial effect on future repeat cesarean deliveries and on integrity of scar for TOLAC. Besides this, the effect on morbidity associated with adhesion formations on GI and other disturbances.

ABDOMINAL CLOSURE

It is by far and large advocated not to close parietal and visceral peritoneum as it is shown to close on its own within 24 hours post-surgery. Nonclosure is associated in several RCTs with less operative time, less fever, reduced hospital stays, and less need for analgesia compared to closure.

Some limited non-level 1 data suggest that closure of the parietal peritoneum may decrease the risk of future adhesion formation; however, this is so far not authenticated. No trials have evaluated technical aspects of fascial closure at CS. The rectus fascia is best closed with a continuous noninterlocking technique.

As this layer is relatively avascular, locking is likely to strangulate the tissue thereby increasing the risk of fascial dehiscence.

A suture material with good tensile strength and the one which is delayed absorbable is preferred choice. Synthetic braided or monofilament sutures are best suited. While closing the fascia, the closure should start at least 1 cm well beyond the margin and the stitches are placed at 1 cm from the previous stitch. Tissue at no point should be strangulated but enough tension is applied to appose the edges and to obliterate the vessels to achieve hemostasis. Suture should be 5–6 mm away from the cut edges of the wound. Too close to the edge and to the previous stitch may increase the risk of dehiscence.

For patients who are at risk of wound disruption, one should use Smead-Jones technique for suturing or interrupted figure-of-eight suturing, both using delayed absorbable monofilament polyglycolic acid. This technique of closure is preferred for vertical incision in high-risk cases. It is essentially far-near or near-far placement of sutures. The suture passes through the lateral side of anterior rectus sheath along with adjacent subcutaneous tissue; then it crosses middle of the incision and takes the middle edge of the opposite side rectus fascia, followed by middle edge on the same side and finally far end of the opposite side along with subcutaneous tissue.

The subcutaneous tissue is closed if it facilitates skin closure or the thickness is more than 2 cm. In which case it is associated with fewer wound complications, such as hematoma, seroma, wound infection or wound separation.[30]

Prophylactic subcutaneous drainage is associated with no additional benefit. It should therefore not be performed routinely.[31,32] If hemostasis is not adequate, there may be a small reason for keeping intra-abdominal or subcutaneous drain but there is no level one evidence which proves its effectiveness.

The transverse CS should be closed with subcuticular suture. Subcuticular closure significantly decreases the risk of wound complications by 57% (from 10.6 to 4.9%) and specifically wound separation (from 7.4 to 1.6%).[33,34] Staple closure is approximately 7 minutes faster than suture closure.[35]

CONCLUSION

Certain practices involving the performance of a CS require to be investigated, to simplify the technique, and to make it less painful for the patient. Adopting proper basic techniques in combination with evidence-based developments involving a number of aspects of care are being suggested. A Joel-Cohen incision, single-layer closure when feasible and nonperitonealization are currently recommended. It is important to exercise caution, whenever a previous CS is being operated. In certain complex cases, it is essential to seek help and involve seniors. In achieving best results, a CS has to be carefully planned and requisite preparations be made with high degree of anticipation.

REFERENCES

1. Peesay M. Nuchal cord and its implications. Matern Health Neonatol Perinatol. 2017;3:28.
2. Rouse DJ, Owen J. Prophylactic caesarean delivery for fetal macrosomia diagnosed by ultrasonography – a Faustian bargain? Am J Obstet Gynecol. 1999;181(2):332-8.
3. Phelan JP, Stine LE, Edwards NB, Clark SL, Horenstein J. The role of external version in the intrapartum management of the transverse lie presentation. Am J Obstet Gynecol. 1985;151(6):724-6.
4. NICE. (2011). Caesarean section. Clinical guideline CG132. [online] Available from: https://www.nice.org.uk/guidance/cg132 [Last accessed January, 2020].
5. Smith JR, Gaanh JM. The incidence of glove puncture during caesarean section. JOG. 1990;10:317-8.
6. Wilkinson C, Enkin MW. Uterine exteriorization versus intraperitoneal repair at caesarean section. Cochrone Database Syst Rev. 2000;(2):CD000085.
7. Cluver C, Novikova N, Hofmeyr GJ, et al. Maternal position during caesarean section for preventing maternal and neonatal complications. Cochrane Database Syst Rev. 2013;28(3):CD007623.
8. Seropian R, Reynolds BM. Wound infections after preoperative depilatory versus razor preparation. Am J Surg. 1971;121(3):251-4.
9. Megann EF, Dodson MK, Ray MA, et al. Preoperative skin preparation and intraoperative pelvic irrigation: impact on post-cesarean endometritis and wound infection. Obs Gynecol. 1993;81:922-5.
10. Mathai M, Hofmeyr GJ. Abdominal surgical incisions in caesarean section. Cochrane Database Syst Rev. 2007;CD004453.
11. Hofmeyr GJ, Mathai M, Shah A, Novikova N. Techniques for caesarean section. Cochrane Database Syst Rev. 2008;(1):CD004662.
12. Berghella V, Baxter JK, Chauhan SP, Evidence-based surgery for caesarean delivery. Am J Obstet Gynecol. 2005;193(5):1607-17.
13. Ayers JW, Morley GW. Surgical incision for caesarean section. Obstet Gynecol. 1987;70(5):706-11.
14. Giacalone PL, Daures JP, Vignal J Herisson C, Hedon B, Laffargue F. Pfannenstiel versus Maylard incision for caesarean delivery: a randomized controlled trial. Obstet Gynecol. 2002;99(5 Pt 1):745-50.
15. Finan MA, Mastrogiannis DS, Spellacy WN. The "Allis" test for easy cesarean delivery. Am J Obstet Gynecol. 1991;164:772-5.

16. Holmgreen G, Sjoholm L, Stark M. The Misgav Ladach method for caesarean section: method description. Acta Obstet Gynecol Scand. 1999;78(7):615-21.
17. Boyle JG, Gabbe SG. T and J vertical extensions in low transverse caesarean births. Obstet Gynecol. 1996;87(2):238-43.
18. Landon MB. Vaginal birth after caesarean delivery. Clin Perinat. 2008;35(3): 491-504.
19. Datta S, Ostheimer GW, Weiss JB, Brown WU Jr, Alper MH. Neonatal effects of prolonged anesthetic induction for caesarean section. Obstet Gynecol. 1981;58(3):331-5.
20. Lurie S, Sulema V, Kohen-Sacher B, Sadan O, Glezerman M. The decision to delivery interval in emergency and non-urgent caesarean sections. Eur J Obstet Gynecol Rep Biol. 2004;113(2):182-5.
21. Arad I, Linder N, Bercovici B. Vacuum extraction at caesarean section – neonatal outcome. J Perinat Med. 1986;14(2):137-40.
22. Magann EF, Dodson MK, Allbert JR, McCurdy CM Jr, Martin RW, Morrison JC. Blood loss at the time of cesarean section by method of placental removal and exteriorization versus in situ repair of uterine incision. Surg Gynecol Obstet. 1993;177(4):389-92.
23. Anorlu RI, Maholwana B, Hofmeyr GJ. Method of delivering the placenta at cesarean section. Cochrane Database Syst Rev. 2008;(3):CD004737.
24. Walsh CA, Walsh SR. Extra-abdominal vs intra-abdominal repair at caesarean delivery: a meta-analysis. Am J Obstet Gynecol. 2009;200(6):625.
25. Dahlke JD, Mendez-Figueroa H, Rouse DJ, Berghella V, Baxter JK, Chauhan SP. Evidence-based surgery for cesarean delivery Am J Obstet Gynecol. 2013;209(4):294-306.
26. Ahmed B, Abu Nahia F, Abushama M. Routine cervical dilatation during elective cesarean section and its influence on maternal morbidity: a randomized controlled study. J Perinat Med. 2005;33(6):510-3.
27. Hohlagschwandtner M, Chalubinski K, Nather A, Husslein P, Joura EA. Continuous v/s interrupted sutures for single layer closure of uterine incision at cesarean section. Arch Gynecol Obstet. 2003;268(1):26-8.
28. Dodd JM, Anderson ER, Gates S, Grivell RM. Surgical techniques for uterine incision and uterine closure at the time of cesarean section. Cochrane Database Syst Rev. 2014;(7).
29. Dodd JM, Anderson ER, Gates S. Surgical techniques for uterine incision and uterine closure at the time of cesarean section. Cochrane Database Syst Rev. 2008;(3):CD004732.
30. Anderson ER, Gates S. Techniques and materials for closure of the abdominal wall in caesarean section. Cochrane Database Syst Review. 2004;(4):CD004663.
31. Gates S, Anderson ER. Wound drainage for caesarean section. Cochrane Database Syst Rev. 2013;(12):CD004549.
32. CAESAR study collaborative group. Caesarean section surgical techniques: a randomized factorial trial (CAESAR). BJOG. 2010;117(11):1366-76.
33. Mackeen AD, Khaifeh K, Fleischer J, Vogell A, Han C, Sendecki J, et al. Suture compared with staple skin closure after cesarean delivery: a randomized controlled trial. Obstet Gynecol. 2014;123(6):1169-75.
34. Mackeen AD, Berghella V, Larsen ML. Techniques and materials for skin closure skin closure in cesarean section. Cochrane Database Syst Rev. 2012;(9):CD003577.
35. Mackeen AD, Schuster M, Berghella V. Suture versus staples for skin closure after cesarean: a metaanalysis. Am J Obstet Gynecol. 2015;212(5):621.

4

Obstetric Hemorrhage

Parag Biniwale, Pankaj Sarode ■

■ INTRODUCTION

Postpartum hemorrhage (PPH) is a treatable obstetric emergency, delayed treatment in which case can result in significant morbidity and mortality. Obstetric hemorrhage still remains the major cause of maternal deaths in developed and developing world. Though obstetric hemorrhage includes bleeding during pregnancy, childbirth, and postpartum, more focus needs to be given to PPH. There is evidence of substandard care in all deaths due to obstetric hemorrhage. The prevention and treatment of PPH are vital steps toward improving the health care of women during childbirth.

Defining PPH is confusing as there are many definitions of it in literature. The one which describes it the best and which is clinically pertinent is the amount of blood loss post-delivery which compromises maternal health due to adverse hemodynamic changes.

Women suffer from complications of pregnancy even when they live in an environment of national prosperity as maternal death can occur in a short period of time due to irreversible shock. Approximately 40% of blood loss at birth is considered as life threatening. Our aim as clinicians should be to arrest the blood loss well below this life-threatening level, generally considered as 1,000 mL. Measurement of blood loss by visual estimation is grossly underestimated. Blood collecting drapes or pictorial estimation may be a better option. It is always better to over diagnose and over treat PPH so that to lose time to start obstetric hemorrhage protocol.

Traditionally, PPH is related to abnormalities of one of the following factors:
- *Tone*—uterine atony/inversion
- *Tissue*—retained bits of placenta/membrane
- *Trauma*—genital trauma, vaginal/cervical tears, rupture uterus
- *Thrombin*—abnormalities of coagulation.

Most cases of PPH have no identifiable risk factors. Still, a few associated factors, which predispose women for PPH, can be identified during antepartum and intrapartum period.

Antenatal factors include:
- Suspected or proven placental abruption
- Known placenta previa

- Abnormally adherent placenta (placenta accreta or increta or percreta)
- *Overdistended uterus*: Multiple pregnancy, polyhydramnios
- Pre-eclampsia/gestational hypertension
- Grand multiparity
- Pre-existing bleeding disorders such as hemophilia
- Treatment with anticoagulants.

Intrapartum factors include:
- Delivery by emergency/elective cesarean section
- Retained placenta
- Episiotomy
- Operative vaginal delivery
- Prolonged labor (>12 h)
- Big baby (>4 kg)
- Pyrexia in labor
- Induction of labor.

Postpartum hemorrhage (PPH) may be aggravated by pre-existing factors such as obesity, anemia, and hypertension. Women with PPH in previous delivery have five times more chance of PPH in subsequent delivery.

More women without risk factors have atonic PPH compared to those with risk factors. Hence, intervention should be targeted at all women during childbirth to prevent uterine atony which is the leading cause of PPH. Active management of third stage of labor (AMTSL) lowers maternal blood loss and lowers the risk of PPH (Cochrane reviews of 2000 and 2011).[1,2] According to WHO, three essential components of AMTSL are:
- Oxytocin-given prophylactically can reduce 60% risk of PPH. It should be given in the dose of 10 IU IV infusion or 5U IM.
  Intramuscular administration should be avoided in case of cardiovascular disorders. Oral misoprostol is not as effective as oxytocin for AMTSL but can be used if oxytocin is not available or trained healthcare worker is not available. It has an advantage of ease of administration and it does not require special storage conditions.
- Controlled cord traction
- Uterine message after delivery of placenta.

Once PPH sets in, management involves:
- Communication
- Resuscitation
- Monitoring and investigations
- Arresting further blood loss

All the above components need to be executed simultaneously.

The following initial assessment and basic treatment should be instituted:
- Call for help
- Assess airway, breathing, and circulation (ABC)

- Provide supplementary oxygen (10–15 L/min regardless of oxygen saturation)
- Obtain an intravenous line (16/18 gauge)
- Start fluid replacement with intravenous crystalloid fluid (at least 3.5 L warmed fluids)
- Monitor blood pressure, pulse and respiration and temperature
- Catheterize bladder and monitor urinary output
- Assess need for blood transfusion
- Order laboratory tests—complete blood count, coagulation screen, blood grouping, and cross-match
- Start intravenous oxytocin infusion.

COMMUNICATION

Principle: Multidisciplinary involvement and transparent communication with relatives.

Ask for help and do call in other senior gynecologists, anesthetists, and physicians for help immediately, as PPH needs multidisciplinary approach. Inform blood bank and laboratory about possibility of need for massive transfusion.

Most important part, which is often neglected, is to communicate with birth attendant and close relative giving them clear idea about severity of the situation. This should be done preferably by a senior and responsible team member and preferably the same person should keep on updating them about the situation intermittently.

RESUSCITATION

Principle: Replacement of blood volume over shortest possible time and restoration of cell perfusion by increasing oxygen carrying capacity.[3,4]

Fluid resuscitation in women with PPH is overly conservative due to underestimated loss, women compensating easily due to hypervolemia of pregnancy, fear of pulmonary edema and failure to appreciate the dynamic fluid shifts in body. Start infusion of crystalloids as soon as PPH is diagnosed. Normal saline or Lactated Ringer's solution is preferred. Normal saline is a reasonable choice as it is compatible with most drugs and blood transfusion. *Dextrose-containing solutions have no role in management of PPH.*

Approximately three times the volume of blood lost needs to be replaced rapidly using crystalloids as infused fluid is not retained in intravascular compartment but instead shifts to interstitial compartment.

Randomized controlled trials have shown that use of colloids have 11 times higher mortality as compared to crystalloids when used for resuscitation. Also, colloids are known to interfere with hemostasis.

▓ MONITORING AND INVESTIGATIONS

Principle: Ongoing assessment of cardiorespiratory status and investigations to assess status of coagulation function.

A quick baseline measurement of pulse, blood pressure, oxygen saturation, and urine output should be done. The parameters need to be measured at frequent intervals to assess the response to treatment.

▓ ARRESTING OF BLOOD LOSS

Principle: To stop blood loss to avoid deterioration of shock condition.

Empty bladder by inserting an indwelling catheter. Massage the uterus bimanually, one hand in vagina in posterior fornix and other one on the abdomen covering fundus, as soon as PPH is suspected. One can compress the uterus and keep it compressed till further help arrives or till the patient is settled down. Aortic compression till definite surgical therapy is executed or during transportation to higher center is life-saving. All these methods help by arresting further blood loss by mechanical pressure.

If available, nonpneumatic antishock garment for temporary maintenance of circulation can be used, till definite treatment is executed.

Uterine packing, considered to be effective in the past, should not be done.

If messaging and compression are found to be ineffective, surgical management protocol needs to be executed. Till the arrangements for surgical interventions are done, following pharmacological measures should be tried:

- *Oxytocin 20–40 IU in infusion*: It can be allowed to run free till bleeding stops then 125 mL/h. One should not administer more than 3 L of IV fluids containing oxytocin as it may cause profound hypotension.
- *Ergometrine 0.2 mg preferably intramuscularly*: It can be repeated every 15 minutes for five doses, if needed. Care should be taken in women with severe hypertension and heart disease.
- *Carboprost 0.25 mg IM every 15 minutes for maximum eight doses*: It may be given intra-myometrialy, although it is an off label use.
  It is not meant for IV administration and should be avoided in women with asthma.
- *Misoprostol 600–1,000 μg*: It can be administered sublingually/rectally/buccally/vaginally. It helps to cause sustained uterine contraction and helps avoid recurrence of uterine atony.

▓ SURGICAL MEASURES

Balloon Tamponade

It is the first line surgical management for uterine atony using Foley's catheter, Bakri balloon. Sengstaken-Blakemore esophageal catheter, condom catheter, or surgical glove tamponade. If bleeding is not arrested then laparotomy is

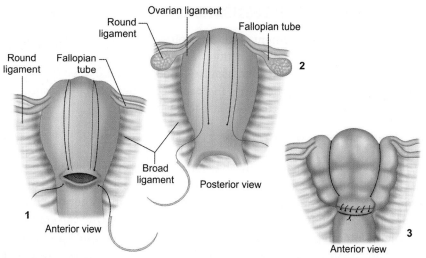

Fig. 1: Parts (1) and (2) describe the anterior and posterior views of the uterus showing the process of the B-Lynch Brace suture. Part (3) shows the anatomical appearance after the suturing.

needed. If bleeding stops then tamponade removal can be planned in 6 h but should be preferably planned at daytime when competent personnel and infrastructure is available to handle the bleeding if it recurs. Balloon may be deflated gradually and may be left in place for some more time to avoid sudden deflation and recurrence of bleeding.

Brace Sutures

The best known version, described by B-Lynch in 1997, requires hysterotomy for its insertion and is particularly suitable when the uterus has already been opened at cesarean section **(Fig. 1)**.[5] A modified compression suture that does not require hysterotomy was described by Hayman et al. in 2002. Other authors, Hwu et al., 2005 and Kafali et al., 2003 have described variants on these techniques. There is no comparative data to demonstrate that any one variant is superior to other. It is recommended that a laminated diagram of the brace technique should be kept in theater. Possible complications of the technique include pyometra and partial uterine necrosis.

Stepwise Devascularization

If bleeding is still not arrested then stepwise devascularization may be needed. Following vessels are ligated in succession to decrease blood flow to uterus.

Uterine vessels are ligated bilaterally. Remember to take a chunk of adjacent uterine musculature in the ligature while doing it. Bilateral ovarian vessels are ligated next, taking care not to obliterate Fallopian tubes. This may not be completely effective due to extensive collateral circulation supplying the uterus. It may not work especially in cases of placenta previa or trauma to lower segment of uterus.

In that case, bilateral internal iliac ligation should be considered. This procedure is time consuming and potentially complicated due to need for retroperitoneal dissection. It should be attempted only if an experienced, senior surgeon is available. Otherwise, no time should be wasted to proceed to obstetric hysterectomy.

One should not delay a decision to perform hysterectomy in view of preserving fertility of the woman.

Obstetric Hysterectomy

Hysterectomy may be needed if all conservative surgical procedures fail. It should not be delayed till woman is exsanguinated and is in irreversible shock. If the operating surgeon has no experience in conservative surgical procedure, then no time should be wasted in attempting them rather than going ahead with hysterectomy. Subtotal hysterectomy is also justified due to its ease of performing and as it consumes less time. But subtotal hysterectomy will not help if it is done in case of cervical trauma or lower segment bleeding as in placenta previa.

Selective Arterial Occlusion (Embolization)

In places where interventional radiology is available and the rate of bleeding allows some time to perform it before irreversible shock sets in. It is of immense help if done before C section for patients with morbidly adherent placentae diagnosed antenatally on ultrasound and confirmed by MRI.

Anesthesia consultant involvement and rapid anesthesia assessment is helpful even when surgical intervention deferred as fluid resuscitation is better guided by a devoted intensivist and *obstetricians* and better focused on arresting blood loss. In case of surgical intervention, regional anesthesia should be avoided in preference for general anesthesia as blood pressure control is better with general anesthesia (GA).

A few tips for safe GA during such emergent situation are:
- Rapid sequence intubation to avoid aspiration
- Cardiostable induction agents with minimal peripheral vasoconstrictor effect
- Adrenaline and atropine availability at induction
- Ventilation with high oxygen concentration, at least till bleeding is arrested.

Avoiding Litigation in PPH

A few tips to avoid future litigation in PPH cases are:
- Communication with relatives by a senior team member, giving them clear idea about possible consequences in an empathetic language.

Documentation of the protocol followed as in the chart below:[6]

Obstetric hemorrhage

Time of call-out:.................... Call-out by:.................... Date: ....

Team member	Name	Time arrived
On-call obstetric consultant		
On-call obstetric senior registrar		
On-call obstetric SpR		
On-call obstetric SHO		
On-call anaesthetic consultant		
On-call anaesthetic senior consultant		
On-call anaesthetic registrar		
On-call operating dept practitioner		
Laboratory technician in haematology		
On-call gynaecology SHO		
Midwife		
Midwife		
Porter		
Cell saver technician		

Drug	Dose	Time
Syntometrine	1 amp IM	
Ergometrine	500 µg/1 amp (if normal BP) IM/IV	
Syntocinon (an MOH trolley or fridge)	40 units in 500 ml physiological saline IV via IVAC pump at 125 ml	
Carboprost	250 µg/1 amp IM	
Carboprost	250 µg/1 amp IM	
Carboprost	250 µg/1 amp IM	
Carboprost	250 µg/1 amp IM	
Carboprost	250 µg/1 amp IM	
Carboprost	250 µg/1 amp IM	
Carboprost	250 µg/1 amp IM	
Misoprostol	200 µg x 5 tablets rectally	

Blood sent	Time	Observations		
		Time	Pulse	B/P
FBC				
Crossmatch units				
Clotting				
Placenta delivered Yes☐ No☐				
Urinary catheter with urimeter				
Fluids				
Type	Volume	Time		

Initial management	Time
Oxygen given	
Head bed down	
Venflons No. 1	
Venflons No. 2	

(Adapted from Chelsea and Westminster Hospital Haemorrhage pro forma)

RCOG Green-top Guideline No. 52

24 of 24

APPENDIX I: Example of a postpartum haemorrhage chart

(It can be done later once the emergency situation is controlled.)
- Following evidence-based management protocols
- Timely transfer to higher centers capable of handling such cases. (Patient can be transferred once life-saving surgical procedure is done and patient is stabilized enough for safe transfer).

■ REFERENCES

1. Mathai M, Gilmezoglu A, Hills S. WHO Department of making pregnancy safer. Recommendations for the prevention of PPH. 2007. Available from: http://www.maternoinfantil.org/archivos/A42.PDF. WHO/MPS/07.06
2. Lewis G. Why mothers die 2000-2002, the sixth report of the confidential enquiries into maternal death in the UK. London: Royal College of Obstetricians and Gynaecologists; 2004.
3. Arulkumaran S, Karoshi M, Keith LG, Lalonde AB, B-Lynch C. A Textbook of Postpartum Hemorrhage, A Comprehensive Guide to Evaluation, Management, and Surgical Intervention. London: Sapiens Publishing.
4. El-Mowafi, DM. (2019). Complications of the third stage of labour, postpartum hemorrhage. [online] Available from: https://www.gfmer.ch/Obstetrics_simplified/postpartum_haemorrhage.htm. [Last accessed January, 2020].
5. Barbieri RL. A stitch in time: the B-Lynch, Hayman, and Pereira uterine compression. OBG Manag. 2012;24(12):6-11.
6. Chelsea and Westminster hospital, post partum hemorrhage proforma.

5   Diabetes in Pregnancy

Pratik Tambe, Ameya Purandare

▇ INTRODUCTION

According to the National Center for Health Statistics (2013), the number of adults diagnosed with diabetes in the United States has tripled from 6.9 million in 1991 to 20.9 million in 2011.[1] Reasons for this rise include an aging population more likely to develop type 2 diabetes, increases in minority groups at particular risk for type 2 diabetes, and dramatic increases in obesity; also referred to as diabesity.

There is keen interest in events that precede diabetes, and this includes the uterine environment, where early imprinting is believed to have effects later in life.[2] For example, in utero exposure to maternal hyperglycemia leads to fetal hyperinsulinemia, causing an increase in fetal fat cells. This leads to obesity and insulin resistance in childhood. This in turn leads to impaired glucose tolerance (IGT) and diabetes in adulthood.[3]

▇ BACKGROUND

Gestational diabetes mellitus (GDM) is defined as impaired glucose tolerance which is first recognized during pregnancy. Worldwide, 10% pregnancies are associated with diabetes and 90% of these cases are GDM.[4] Gestational diabetes which can be treated with diet and exercise therapy alone is termed diet-controlled GDM or class A1GDM. On the other hand, those patients who require medication are referred to as class A2GDM.

The prevalence of GDM varies depending on the prevalence of type 2 diabetes in any population. While Caucasian women have a lower risk, other ethnicities including South Asian women exhibit a higher risk. Gestational diabetes increases with body mass index (BMI) and age. With a preponderance of sedentary lifestyle, the prevalence of GDM worldwide is increasing.[5-6]

In India, prevalence is estimated to be around 10–14.3%, which is much higher than in western countries. As of 2010, there were an estimated 22 million women with diabetes between the ages of 20 and 39 years and an additional 54 million women with IGT who have the potential to develop GDM. This incidence is expected to rise to 20% in the near future.

A study in Tamil Nadu state, the Diabetes in Pregnancy Awareness and Prevention project, found that of 4,151 (urban), 3,960 (semiurban), and 3,945 (rural) pregnant women screened, the prevalence of GDM was 17.8% (urban), 13.8% (semiurban), and 9.9% (rural) areas, respectively.[4]

To address the urgent need to prevent and minimize maternal and fetal morbidity associated with GDM, the Ministry of Health and Family Welfare has released a national guideline for provision of universal screening and management of GDM as part of the essential antenatal package in February 2018.[4]

OBSTETRIC IMPLICATIONS AND LONG-TERM CONSEQUENCES

Maternal risks include polyhydramnios, prolonged and obstructed labor, uterine atony, postpartum hemorrhage, puerperal infection, and progression of diabetic retinopathy. GDM confers a higher risk of preeclampsia (9.8% and 18%, respectively in populations with a fasting glucose <115 mg/dL and >115 mg/dL). Much higher rates of cesarean delivery have been reported (25% of A2GDM and 17% of A1GDM vs. 9.5% in controls).[7] The long-term implications postpregnancy include an increased risk of developing frank diabetes which is influenced by race, ethnicity, and obesity. As much as 70% of women presenting with GDM develop diabetes 2–3 decades later.[8] The risk of progression is highest in Latin American women; as high as 60% within 5 years.[9]

Fetal risks include miscarriage, congenital malformations, and intrauterine fetal death. Neonates born typically exhibit an increased risk of macrosomia, shoulder dystocia, operative vaginal delivery, birth trauma, stillbirth, respiratory distress syndrome, neonatal hypoglycemia, and hyperbilirubinemia. The Hyperglycemia and Adverse Pregnancy Outcome (HAPO) study, reaffirmed the relationship between maternal glucose levels higher birth weights, cesarean delivery, fetal hyperinsulinemia, and neonatal hypoglycemia.[10] Fetal exposure in utero also is an independent risk factor for childhood and adult obesity predisposing to diabetes in the offspring.[11]

SCREENING AND DIAGNOSIS

Previously, the approach to screening for GDM included obtaining a detailed history with focus on past obstetric history, with an emphasis on miscarriages, stillbirths, and details pinpointing labor issues and operative vaginal delivery or shoulder dystocia. A family history of type 2 diabetes was sought. The most widely used screening test in the US (over 95% obstetricians) is the 50-g, 1-hour oral glucose tolerance test (OGTT) which was proposed nearly 50 years ago.[12]

Using only the history, urine sugar, and obesity to identify GDM has a huge potential for failure as approximately 50% of women will be missed. Hence, the US Preventive Services Task Force in 2014 has recommended universal screening for all pregnant women for GDM at or beyond 24 weeks of gestation.[13]

SCREENING METHODOLOGIES

Universal screening is usually performed at 24–28 weeks of gestation. Early pregnancy screening for undiagnosed type 2 diabetes may include a fasting blood glucose followed by a 75-g glucose load and a 2-hour plasma glucose measurement. Many obstetricians use the two-step screening process that is used for GDM and start with a 50-g OGTT.[13]

The American Diabetes Association (ADA) recommends that HbA_{1C} may not be suitable for use alone because of decreased sensitivity compared with the OGTT.[14] GDM screening is still to be performed at 24–28 weeks in women who have negative early pregnancy screening.

Two-step Approach

Some obstetricians like to follow a two-step approach. This involves first screening with the administration of a 50-g oral glucose load and a 1-hour venous glucose sample. Women whose glucose levels exceed the screening threshold (130 or 140 mg/dL) then undergo a formal 100-g, 3-hour diagnostic OGTT. GDM is diagnosed when there are two or more abnormal values on the 3-hour OGTT. There is a lack of consensus for a universal cutoff value. There is currently insufficient data regarding the ideal cutoff value in order to improve pregnancy outcomes.[15-17]

3-hour OGTT

Table 1 sets out the threshold values in mg/dL and mmol/L for the 3-hour OGTT by the National Diabetes Data Group and by Carpenter and Coustan. The latter uses more strict values resulting in improved rates of diagnosis.[14,18] Women who have even one abnormal value with a formal 100-g, 3-hour OGTT have a significantly increased risk of adverse perinatal outcomes compared to controls.[19]

TABLE 1: Proposed diagnostic criteria for gestational diabetes mellitus.*				
	Plasma or serum glucose level Carpenter and Coustan conversion		Plasma level national diabetes data group conversion	
Status	mg/dL	mmol/L	mg/dL	mmol/L
Fasting	95	5.3	105	5.8
1 hour	180	10.0	190	10.6
2 hours	155	8.6	165	9.2
3 hours	140	7.8	145	8.0

*A diagnosis generally requires that two or more thresholds be met or exceeded, although some clinicians choose to use just one elevated value.
Source: Adapted with permission from the American Diabetes Association. Classification and Diagnosis of Diabetes. Diabetes Care. 2017;40(Suppl 1):S11-24.

A single-step single-value approach using a 75-g, 2-hour OGTT has been used and promoted. In 2010, the International Association of Diabetes and Pregnancy Study Group (IADPSG) has recommended a universal 75-g, 2-hour OGTT be performed during pregnancy and that the diagnosis of GDM be established when any single threshold value was met or exceeded (fasting value 92 mg/dL; 1 hour value 180 mg/dL; or 2 hour value 153 mg/dL). These criteria would identify approximately 18% of pregnant women in the United States as having GDM and in other subpopulations, the incidence would be even higher.[20]

In 2011, the ADA endorsed these criteria while acknowledging that adopting these cutoffs would significantly increase the prevalence of GDM. The additional women in whom GDM would be diagnosed may be at a lower risk of adverse outcomes and may not derive similar benefits from diagnosis and treatment as women in whom GDM was diagnosed by traditional criteria. As of 2017, the ADA recognizes that there is an absence of clear evidence that supports the IADPSG recommended approach versus the more traditional two-step screening approach.[20]

SUMMARY OF RECOMMENDATIONS ON SCREENING

The Eunice Kennedy Shriver National Institute of Child Health and Human Development Consensus Development Conference on Diagnosing Gestational Diabetes (2013) recommended that obstetricians continue to use a two-step approach.[15,21] A Cochrane review (2015) supported that no specific screening strategy has been shown to be optimal.[22] Hence, the American College of Obstetricians and Gynecologists (ACOG) supports the two-step process.[23]

The National Institute for Health and Care Excellence (NICE) and Australian guidelines recommend a risk-based screening with 75 g, 2 hours OGTT with fasting blood sugar ≥126 mg/dL and 2 hours ≥140 mg/dL taken as diagnostic for GDM. The World Health Organization (WHO) and The International Federation of Gynecology and Obstetrics (FIGO) endorse universal screening for GDM at 24–28 weeks of gestation using the 75 g with 2 hours glucose (fasting ≥126 mg/dL and ≥140 mg/dL). Studies in India conducted by Federation of Obstetric and Gynecological Societies of India (FOGSI) and Diabetes in Pregnancy Study Group in India (DIPSI) endorse the "Single-step single-value test" with cut-off 2 hours 75 g post blood sugar ≥140 mg/dL being simple, accurate, and economical **(Flowchart 1)**.[4]

BENEFITS OF INSTITUTING TREATMENT

The Australian Carbohydrate Intolerance Study in Pregnant Women (ACHOIS) trial (2005) on 1,000 women found that treatment was associated with a significant reduction in the rate of serious newborn complications such as perinatal death, shoulder dystocia, birth trauma, fracture, and nerve palsy.

Flowchart 1: Screening pathways—GOI guidelines.[4]

Universal testing for GDM

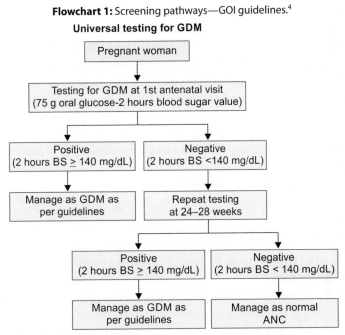

(BS: blood sugar; GDM: gestational diabetes mellitus; ANC: antenatal care)

There was a reduction in risk of preeclampsia (18–12%), reduction in large-for-gestational-age (LGA) babies (22–13%), and birth weights >4 kg (21–10%).[24]

A subsequent trial of 958 women with mild GDM in the United States found no differences in the frequency of perinatal deaths, neonatal hypoglycemia, elevated umbilical cord C-peptide level, and birth trauma. However, significant differences in secondary outcomes were observed with treatment including lower rates of cesarean section, shoulder dystocia, preeclampsia, lower frequency of LGA infants, lower frequency of birth weight exceeding 4 kg, and reduced neonatal fat mass.[21]

A US Preventive Services Task Force systematic review has emphasized these benefits.[25] The treatment offered is specific dietary counseling and exercise.[26-27] When this fails, medication should be instituted. In both these trials, women refractory to medical nutrition therapy were treated with insulin and not oral agents.

■ MONITORING RESPONSE TO THERAPY

Periodic blood glucose testing is required in patients who institute medical nutrition therapy. However, there is insufficient evidence to define the frequency at which such testing should take place. The general recommendation is monitoring four times a day, once after fasting and again after each meal.

Fasting glucose values are predictive of increased neonatal fat mass and hence may be useful in monitoring. A randomized controlled trial comparing preprandial versus postprandial measurements has shown that a 1-hour postprandial measurement was associated with better glycemic control, a lower incidence of LGA infants and lower cesarean section rates. Hence, fasting and postprandial values may be used for monitoring.[28]

The ADA and ACOG both recommend that fasting blood glucose values should be <95 mg/dL and postprandial blood glucose values should be <140 mg/dL at 1 hour or <120 mg/dL at 2 hours to reduce the risk of macrosomia.[14]

ROLE OF DIET AND EXERCISE

Nonpharmacological approaches of dietary modification, exercise, and glucose monitoring form the first-line approach. A Cochrane meta-analysis of lifestyle modification trials in women with GDM demonstrated benefit with a reduction in LGA neonates, macrosomia (baby weight >4 kg), and neonatal fat mass **(Table 2)**.[29]

The goal of medical nutrition therapy in women with GDM is to achieve normal blood glucose levels, prevent ketosis, provide adequate weight gain, and contribute to appropriate fetal growth and development. The ADA recommends nutritional counseling by a registered dietician and a personalized nutrition plan based on the patient's BMI **(Table 3)**.

Carbohydrate intake should be restricted to 33–40% of calories, with the remaining calories divided between protein (20%) and fat (40%). Complex carbohydrates are recommended over simple carbohydrates because they are digested more slowly, are less likely to produce significant postprandial hyperglycemia, and potentially reduce insulin resistance.[30] In practice, three

TABLE 2: Caloric requirements in pregnancy.[4]

	Level of activity	Energy requirement during pregnancy	Total energy requirement (kcal/day)
1.	Sedentary work	1,900 + 350	2,250
2.	Moderate work	2,230 + 350	2,580
3.	Heavy work	2,850 + 350	3,200

TABLE 3: Caloric requirements as per body mass index (BMI).[4]

Weight category	BMI (kg/m²)	Energy requirement (kcal/day)
Underweight	<18.5	Energy requirement as per level of activity + 500 kcal/day
Normal weight	18.5–22.9	Energy requirement as per level of activity
Overweight	23–24.9	Energy requirement as per level of activity
Obese	>25	Energy requirement as per level of activity – 500 kcal/day

meals and two to three snacks are recommended to distribute carbohydrate intake and to reduce postprandial glucose fluctuations.

Individualization is important when determining energy requirement, and adjustments should be made based on weight change patterns. Energy requirement during pregnancy includes the normal requirement of adult and an additional requirement for fetal growth plus the increase in the body weight of pregnant woman. Energy requirement does not increase in the first trimester unless a woman is underweight; it increases during second and third trimester.

Energy intake should be adequate enough to provide appropriate weight gain during pregnancy. As per the Indian Council of Medical Research (ICMR) guidelines, for an average weight gain of 10–12 kg, an addition of 350 kcal/day above the adult requirement is recommended during second and third trimester. Severe caloric restriction is not recommended as it may result in ketonemia and ketonuria and impair physical and mental development in offspring.[4]

There are few published exercise trials in women with GDM which have small sample sizes and they appear to show improvement in glucose levels.[31] In nonpregnant diabetic women, weight training increases lean muscle mass and improves tissue sensitivity to insulin. In GDM accompanied by high BMI, exercise may be able to improve glycemic control and moderate exercise is recommended as part of the treatment plan. Women with GDM should aim for 30 minutes of moderate-intensity aerobic exercise at least 5 days a week or a minimum of 150 minutes per week. Even walking for 10–15 minutes after a meal can lead to better glycemic control and is commonly recommended.[32]

■ PHARMACOLOGICAL TREATMENT

Insulin

Insulin is the gold standard therapy for GDM management in patients refractory to medical nutrition and exercise therapy. It is generally started if fasting blood glucose levels are ≥95 mg/dL, if 1 hour levels are ≥140 mg/dL, or if 2 hours levels are ≥120 mg/dL **(Flowchart 2)**.

The typical starting total dosage is 0.7–1.0 units/kg body weight daily. This dosage can be divided amongst multiple injections using long-acting or intermediate-acting insulin in combination with short-acting insulin. If there are isolated abnormal values at specific times during the day, the insulin regimen should focus on correcting the specific hyperglycemia. When there are elevated fasting values, previous night administration of intermediate-acting insulin may be adequate. In women with elevated values only at breakfast or postprandially, short-acting insulin before breakfast is appropriate.

Alternatives to neutral protamine Hagedorn insulin (NPH), such as glargine and insulin detemir, are prescribed for long-acting use. Insulin analogs lispro and aspart have a more rapid onset of action, enabling

Flowchart 2: Insulin therapy pathways.[4]

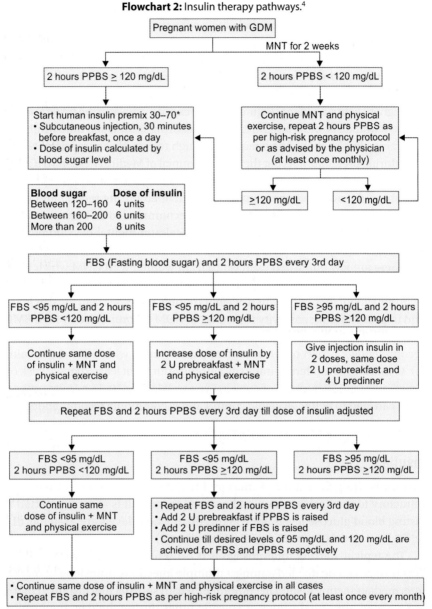

*Only injection human premix insulin 30/70 to be used
* Insulin syringe–40 IU syringe * Subcutaneous injection only

(GDM: gestational diabetes mellitus; MNT: medical nutrion therapy; PPBS: postprandial blood sugar)

the patient to administer her insulin at the time of a meal rather than 10–15 minutes earlier. This provides better glycemic control and helps avoid hypoglycemic episodes.

Oral Antidiabetics

Despite them not being approved by the US Food and Drug Administration (FDA) for this purpose, oral antidiabetic agents including metformin have been widely used for treatment of women with GDM. Insulin is the recommended modality as per the ADA.

Metformin belongs to the class of biguanides and inhibits hepatic gluconeogenesis, glucose absorption, and stimulates glucose uptake in peripheral tissues. Metformin has been extensively used in gynecological practice in women with IGT or more commonly in polycystic ovary syndrome and fertility issues. The usual dosage for metformin is 500 mg nightly for 1 week initially and then increases to 500 mg twice or thrice daily.

In women with polycystic ovary syndrome (PCOS), metformin is commonly continued throughout the first trimester, which is not an evidence-based practice. There is scant evidence to suggest that metformin decreases the risks of miscarriage.[33] Unlike insulin, metformin crosses the placenta and levels that can be as high as maternal peripheral blood concentrations. The long-term metabolic influence of such levels on the offspring is as yet unknown.[34] In view of this, the ADA recommends that in pharmacological treatment of GDM, insulin should be considered the drug of choice.

Metformin versus Insulin Therapy

A meta-analysis of published data revealed that the differences between neonates delivered by women randomized to metformin versus insulin were minimal.[35-36] Women administered metformin experienced a higher rate of preterm birth [risk ratio (RR) 1.5]. A more recent meta-analysis did not demonstrate superiority when metformin was compared with insulin on neonatal outcomes.[37]

Hence, although metformin is being used to treat GDM, patients must be counseled about the lack of equivalence with insulin, the issues of placental transfer, and the absence of data regarding long-term effects on exposed offspring. Almost half of all patients on metformin eventually require insulin.[38] In women who decline insulin therapy, cannot afford it or who are unable to regularly administer it, metformin may be a reasonable alternative choice.

Glyburide

Glyburide belongs to the class of sulfonylureas and binds to pancreatic beta-cell adenosine triphosphate potassium channel receptors to increase insulin secretion and insulin sensitivity of peripheral tissues. Meta-analyses have noted increased risks of macrosomia and hypoglycemia with glyburide compared with insulin in the treatment of GDM[37] whereas a more recent meta-analysis only demonstrated higher rates of neonatal hypoglycemia.[39] Glyburide should not be recommended as it does not yield equivalent outcomes to insulin or metformin. Safety during pregnancy is also a matter of concern.

FETAL ASSESSMENT

Antepartum fetal testing is recommended for patients with IGT. There is an increased risk of fetal demise in patients with IGT related to suboptimal glycemic control. Similarly, women with GDM who have poor glycemic control are also at an increased risk. Fetal surveillance may be beneficial for patients with GDM exhibiting poor glycemic control.

Antenatal fetal testing is usually initiated at 32 weeks of gestation. If multiple other factors associated with increased risk of adverse pregnancy outcome are present, surveillance may start earlier. Studies have not demonstrated an increase in adverse outcomes in A1GDM patients before 40 weeks of gestation and increased antepartum fetal testing may not be necessary in these women.

There is no consensus regarding antepartum fetal testing among A1GDM patients. If required, it is generally started later than in women with A2GDM. There are no standard recommendations regarding the specific antepartum test and frequency of testing. These may be as per local institutional policies and obstetrician preferences. However, since polyhydramnios is an important outcome, it is common for clinicians to measure amniotic fluid volume serially.

TIMING AND MODE OF DELIVERY

Patients with well-controlled GDM and no complications can be managed expectantly until term.[40] In most cases, women with good glycemic control who are receiving medical therapy (A2GDM) do not require delivery before 39 weeks of gestation. Since fetal lung maturity is delayed in GDM, dexamethasone may be administered as appropriate and delivery before 39 weeks avoided in well-controlled patients except when there are other complications.

The GINEXMAL trial where patients were randomized to induction of labor at 38 weeks versus expectant management up to 41 weeks of gestation showed no difference in cesarean delivery rates (12.6% vs. 11.8%, $p = 0.81$) or many other outcomes. Neonatal hyperbilirubinemia was more common in the induced group (10.0% vs. 4.1%, $p = 0.03$).[41]

In a randomized trial women with A2GDM and AGA fetuses were randomized at 38 weeks of gestation to induction of labor within 1 week or expectant management; there was no difference in cesarean section rates.[42] The proportion of LGA infants was smaller in the induction group.

There are no significant differences in either macrosomia or cesarean section rates among women with insulin-treated GDM who underwent induction of labor at 38–39 weeks of gestation when compared with expectantly managed controls.[43] Shoulder dystocia was experienced by 10% of the expectant management group after more than 40 weeks of gestation versus 1.4% in the group with labor induction at 38–39 weeks of gestation.

Delivery in women with A1GDM should not be before 39 weeks of gestation, unless otherwise indicated. In such women, expectant management up to 40 6/7 weeks of gestation in the setting of indicated antepartum testing is generally appropriate. For women with A2GDM that is well controlled, delivery is recommended from 39 0/7 to 39 6/7 weeks of gestation.

Earlier delivery for women with poorly controlled GDM is a universal recommendation.[40] However, recommendations about the timing of delivery are unclear. The risks of prematurity and the risks of stillbirth need to be balanced. Delivery between 37 0/7 and 38 6/7 weeks of gestation may be justified, but delivery in the late preterm period from 34 0/7 to 36 6/7 weeks of gestation should be reserved for those patients who do not respond to supervised in-hospital treatment or who have abnormal antepartum fetal testing results.

■ MANAGEMENT IN LABOR

Pregnant women with GDM on medical management (metformin or insulin) require blood sugar monitoring during labor by a glucometer. The morning dose of insulin is withheld on the day of induction/labor and the woman should be started on 2 hourly monitoring of blood sugar. Intravenous (IV) infusion with normal saline (NS) to be started and regular insulin should be added according to blood sugar levels as per **Table 4**.

■ MACROSOMIA AND SHOULDER DYSTOCIA

Macrosomia is more common in women with GDM and shoulder dystocia is more likely at fetal weight in GDM pregnancies when compared to controls. Hence, it is recommended that clinicians assess fetal growth by ultrasonography late in the third trimester and identify macrosomia among women with GDM.[41-42]

TABLE 4: Insulin administration in labor.[4]		
Blood sugar level	*Amount of insulin added in 500 mL NS*	*Rate of NS infusion*
90–120 mg/dL	0	100 mL/h (16 drops/min)
120–140 mg/dL	4 U	100 mL/h (16 drops/min)
140–180 mg/dL	6 U	100 mL/h (16 drops/min)
>180 mg/dL	8 U	100 mL/h (16 drops/min)
(NS: normal saline)		

Although such screening is common, one recent study found that among cases of ultrasonography-diagnosed LGA infants, only 22% were LGA at birth.[43] Studies are inconclusive whether cesarean section should be performed to reduce the risk of birth trauma in cases of suspected macrosomia.

It has been estimated that approximately 588 cesarean deliveries would be needed to prevent a single case of permanent brachial plexus palsy for an estimated fetal weight of 4.5 kg and up to 962 cesarean deliveries would be needed for an estimated fetal weight of 4 kg. It is recommend that women with GDM should be counseled regarding the risks and benefits of a scheduled cesarean delivery when the estimated fetal weight is 4.5 kg or more.[44]

It is beyond the scope of this chapter to discuss the management of shoulder dystocia in detail and the HELPERR pathway is depicted in **Flowchart 3** in brief for reference.

Flowchart 3: HELPERR pathway (RCOG Green-top Guideline on shoulder dystocia).

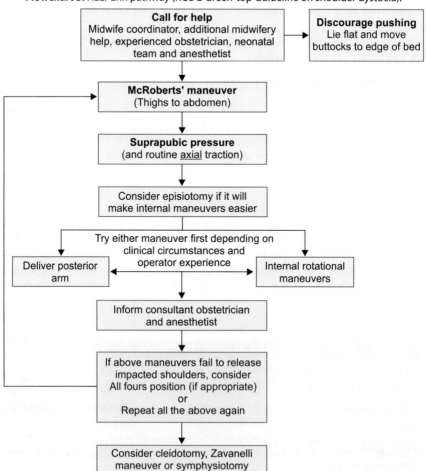

■ POSTPARTUM FOLLOW-UP AND COUNSELING

Generally, carbohydrate intolerance resolves in the postpartum period, but up to one-third of women will have diabetes or IGT at postpartum screening. It has been estimated that between 15 and 70% will develop type 2 diabetes later in life, at varying intervals after the index pregnancy, depending on BMI, race, and ethnicity.[45]

Hence, screening 4–12 weeks postdelivery is recommended for all women with GDM. A fasting plasma glucose test and the 75 g, 2-hour OGTT have both been used for diagnosing overt diabetes in the postpartum period. The Fifth International Workshop on Gestational Diabetes Mellitus has recommended the latter as the preferred method in the postpartum period.[46]

All GDM patients should follow-up with their primary care physician postdelivery. Women with IGT and diabetes should be referred for appropriate preventive or medical therapy. Women with IGT may respond to diet, nutrition, and exercise therapy while patients with frank diabetes will require intensive medical therapy with insulin.

Repeat annual screening at a DM (diabetes millitus) or NCD (noncommunicable disease) clinic is recommended by the ADA, ACOG, and Government of India (GOI) for such with normal postpartum screening test results. Screening between pregnancies can detect abnormal glucose metabolism before conception and can help to ensure good pre-pregnancy glucose levels in subsequent pregnancies. Women should be encouraged to discuss their GDM history and counseled regarding the need for screening during future pregnancies.[47]

■ CONCLUSION

Diabetes during pregnancy is a challenging scenario for obstetricians which requires close monitoring and multidisciplinary care. Ensuring individualization of treatment and carefully tailored approaches at the appropriate juncture can help to enhance the maternal and fetal outcomes. Since this condition is a disease of modern civilization, its incidence is expected to explode in the coming decades. Being armed with the newest evidence and evidence-based recommendations will go a long way toward helping the modern obstetrician deal with such patients.

■ REFERENCES

1. Centers for Disease Control and Prevention (2010). Press release: number of Americans with diabetes projected to double or triple by 2050. October 22, 2010. [online] Available from: http:/www.cdc.gov/media/pressrel/2010/r101022.html [Last accessed on January, 2020].
2. Saudek CD. Progress and promise of diabetes research. JAMA. 2002;287(19):2582-4.
3. Feig DS, Palda VA. Type 2 diabetes in pregnancy: a growing concern. Lancet. 2002;359:1690.

 4. Diagnosis and Management of Gestational Diabetes Mellitus. Technical and Operational Guidelines. Maternal Health Division, Ministry of Health and Family Welfare, Government of India. A GOI-UNICEF Publication. February 2018.
 5. Getahun D, Nath C, Ananth CV, Chavez MR, Smulian JC, et al. Gestational diabetes in the United States: temporal trends 1989 through 2004. Am J Obstet Gynecol. 2008;198:525.e1-5.
 6. Caughey AB, Cheng YW, Stotland NE, Washington AE, Escobar GJ. Maternal and paternal race/ethnicity are both associated with gestational diabetes. Am J Obstet Gynecol. 2010;202:616.e1-5.
 7. England LJ, Dietz PM, Njoroge T, Callaghan WM, Bruce C, Buus RM, et al. Preventing type 2 diabetes: public health implications for women with a history of gestational diabetes mellitus. Am J Obstet Gynecol. 2009;200:365.e1-8.
 8. Kim C, Newton KM, Knopp RH. Gestational diabetes and the incidence of type 2 diabetes: a systematic review. Diabetes Care. 2002;25:1862-8.
 9. Kjos SL, Peters RK, Xiang A, Henry OA, Montoro M, Buchanan TA. Predicting future diabetes in Latino women with gestational diabetes. Utility of early post-partum glucose tolerance testing. Diabetes. 1995;44:586-91.
10. Metzger BE, Lowe LP, Dyer AR, Trimble ER, Chaovarindr U, Coustan DR, et al. Hyperglycemia and adverse pregnancy outcomes. HAPO Study Cooperative Research Group. N Engl J Med. 2008;358:1991-2002.
11. Clausen TD, Mathiesen ER, Hansen T, Pedersen O, Jensen DM, Lauenborg J, et al. Overweight and the metabolic syndrome in adult offspring of women with diet-treated gestational diabetes mellitus or type 1 diabetes. J Clin Endocrinol Metab. 2009;94:2464-70.
12. Gabbe SG, Gregory RP, Power ML, Williams SB, Schulkin J. Management of diabetes mellitus by obstetrician-gynecologists. Obstet Gynecol. 2004;103: 1229-34.
13. Moyer VA; U.S. Preventive Services Task Force. Screening for gestational diabetes mellitus: U.S. Preventive Services Task Force recommendation statement. Ann Intern Med. 2014;160:414-20.
14. American Diabetes Association. Management of diabetes in pregnancy. Diabetes Care. 2017;40:S114-9.
15. Chamberlain JJ, Rhinehart AS, Shaefer CF Jr, Neuman A. Diagnosis and management of diabetes: synopsis of the 2016 American Diabetes Association Standards of Medical Care in Diabetes. Ann Intern Med. 2016;164:542-52.
16. Vandorsten JP, Dodson WC, Espeland MA, Grobman WA, Guise JM, Mercer BM, et al. NIH consensus development conference: diagnosing gestational diabetes mellitus. NIH Consens State Sci Statements. 2013;29:1-31.
17. Esakoff TF, Cheng YW, Caughey AB. Screening for gestational diabetes: different cut-offs for different ethnicities? Am J Obstet Gynecol. 2005;193:1040-4.
18. Ferrara A, Hedderson MM, Quesenberry CP, Selby JV. Prevalence of gestational diabetes mellitus detected by the national diabetes data group or the carpenter and coustan plasma glucose thresholds. Diabetes Care. 2002;25:1625-30.
19. Cheng YW, Block-Kurbisch I, Caughey AB. Carpenter-Coustan criteria compared with the national diabetes data group thresholds for gestational diabetes mellitus. Obstet Gynecol. 2009;114:326-32.
20. Metzger BE, Gabbe SG, Persson B, Buchanan TA, Catalano PA, Damm P, et al. International Association of Diabetes and Pregnancy Study Groups recommendations on the diagnosis and classification of hyperglycemia in pregnancy. International Association of Diabetes and Pregnancy Study Groups Consensus Panel. Diabetes Care. 2010;33:676-82.

21. Landon MB, Spong CY, Thom E, Carpenter MW, Ramin SM, Casey B, et al. A multicenter, randomized trial of treatment for mild gestational diabetes. Eunice Kennedy Shriver National Institute of Child Health and Human Development Maternal-Fetal Medicine Units Network. N Engl J Med. 2009;361:1339-48.
22. American Diabetes Association. Standards of medical care in diabetes—2011. Diabetes Care 2011;34(Suppl 1):S11-61.
23. Farrar D, Duley L, Medley N, Lawlor DA. Different strategies for diagnosing gestational diabetes to improve maternal and infant health. Cochrane Database Syst Rev. 2017;8:CD007122.
24. Crowther CA, Hiller JE, Moss JR, McPhee AJ, Jeffries WS, Robinson JS. Effect of treatment of gestational diabetes mellitus on pregnancy outcomes. Australian Carbohydrate Intolerance Study in Pregnant Women (ACHOIS) Trial Group. N Engl J Med. 2005;352:2477-86.
25. Hartling L, Dryden DM, Guthrie A, Muise M, Vandermeer B, Donovan L. Benefits and harms of treating gestational diabetes mellitus: a systematic review and meta-analysis for the U.S. Preventive Services Task Force and the National Institutes of Health Office of Medical Applications of Research. Ann Intern Med. 2013;159:123-9.
26. Han S, Middleton P, Shepherd E, Van Ryswyk E, Crowther CA. Different types of dietary advice for women with gestational diabetes mellitus. Cochrane Database Syst Rev. 2017;2:CD009275.
27. Barakat R, Pelaez M, Lopez C, Lucia A, Ruiz JR. Exercise during pregnancy and gestational diabetes-related adverse effects: a randomised controlled trial. Br J Sports Med. 2013;47:630-6.
28. de Veciana M, Major CA, Morgan MA, Asrat T, Toohey JS, Lien JM, et al. Postprandial versus preprandial blood glucose monitoring in women with gestational diabetes mellitus requiring insulin therapy. N Engl J Med. 1995;333:1237-41.
29. Brown J, Alwan NA, West J, Brown S, McKinlay CJ, Farrar D, et al. Lifestyle interventions for the treatment of women with gestational diabetes. Cochrane Database Syst Rev. 2017;5:CD011970.
30. Moses RG, Barker M, Winter M, Petocz P, Brand-Miller JC. Can a low-glycemic index diet reduce the need for insulin in gestational diabetes mellitus? A randomized trial. Diabetes Care. 2009;32:996-1000.
31. Ceysens G, Rouiller D, Boulvain M. Exercise for diabetic pregnant women. Cochrane Database Syst Rev. 2006;3:CD004225.
32. Horvath K, Koch K, Jeitler K, Matyas E, Bender R, Bastian H, et al. Effects of treatment in women with gestational diabetes mellitus: systematic review and meta-analysis. BMJ. 2010;340:c1395.
33. De Leo V, Musacchio MC, Piomboni P, Di Sabatino A, Morgante G. The administration of metformin during pregnancy reduces polycystic ovary syndrome related gestational complications. Eur J Obstet Gynecol Reprod Biol. 2011;157:63-6.
34. Wouldes TA, Battin M, Coat S, Rush EC, Hague WM, Rowan JA. Neurodevelopmental outcome at 2 years in offspring of women randomised to metformin or insulin treatment for gestational diabetes. Arch Dis Child Fetal Neonatal Ed. 2016;101:F488-F493.
35. Balsells M, García-Patterson A, Solà I, Roqué M, Gich I, Corcoy R. Glibenclamide, metformin, and insulin for the treatment of gestational diabetes: a systematic review and meta-analysis. BMJ. 2015;350:h102.
36. Poolsup N, Suksomboon N, Amin M. Efficacy and safety of oral antidiabetic drugs in comparison to insulin in treating gestational diabetes mellitus: a meta-analysis. PLoS One. 2014;9:e109985.

37. Farrar D, Simmonds M, Bryant M, Sheldon TA, Tuffnell D, Golder S, et al. Treatments for gestational diabetes: a systematic review and meta-analysis. BMJ Open. 2017;7:e015557.

38. Spaulonci CP, Bernardes LS, Trindade TC, Zugaib M, Francisco RP. Randomized trial of metformin vs insulin in the management of gestational diabetes. Am J Obstet Gynecol. 2013;209:34.e1-7.

39. Song R, Chen L, Chen Y, Si X, Liu Y, Liu Y, et al. Comparison of glyburide and insulin in the management of gestational diabetes: a meta-analysis. PLoS One. 2017;12:e0182488.

40. Medically indicated late-preterm and early-term deliveries. Committee Opinion No. 560. American College of Obstetricians and Gynecologists. Obstet Gynecol. 2013;121:908-10.

41. Alberico S, Erenbourg A, Hod M, Yogev Y, Hadar E, Neri F, et al. Immediate delivery or expectant management in gestational diabetes at term: the GINEXMAL randomised controlled trial. GINEXMAL Group. BJOG. 2017;124:669-77. (Level I)

42. Kjos SL, Henry OA, Montoro M, Buchanan TA, Mestman JH. Insulin-requiring diabetes in pregnancy: a randomized trial of active induction of labor and expectant management. Am J Obstet Gynecol. 1993;169:611-5.

43. Lurie S, Insler V, Hagay ZJ. Induction of labor at 38 to 39 weeks of gestation reduces the incidence of shoulder dystocia in gestational diabetic patients class A2. Am J Perinatol. 1996;13:293-6.

44. American College of Obstetricians and Gynecologists' Committee on Practice Bulletins—Obstetrics. Practice Bulletin No. 173: Fetal macrosomia. Obstet Gynecol. 2016;128(5):e195-209.

45. Chodick G, Elchalal U, Sella T, Heymann AD, Porath A, Kokia E, et al. The risk of overt diabetes mellitus among women with gestational diabetes: a population-based study. Diabet Med. 2010;27:779-85.

46. Metzger BE, Buchanan TA, Coustan DR, de Leiva A, Dunger DB, Hadden DR, et al. Summary and recommendations of the Fifth International Workshop-Conference on Gestational Diabetes Mellitus. Diabetes Care. 2007; (30 Suppl 2):S251-60.

47. Committee on Practice Bulletins—Obstetrics. ACOG Practice Bulletin Number 190: Gestational Diabetes Mellitus. Obstet Gynecol. 2018;131(2):e49-64.

6   Polycystic Ovary Syndrome

N Sanjeeva Reddy, Radha Vembu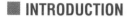

■ INTRODUCTION

Polycystic ovarian syndrome (PCOS) was first described by Irving F Stein and Michael L Leventhal in 1935. It can be found in up to a third of normal cycling or ovulatory women.[1] It is due to functional derangement and not due to any specific central or local defect.

■ DIAGNOSTIC CRITERIA

Polycystic ovarian syndrome is not a specific endocrine disease but it is a syndrome with collection of signs and symptoms and no single sign, symptom or test is diagnostic **(Tables 1 and 2)**.

TABLE 1: Diagnostic criteria for PCOS.

Criteria	NIH 1990	Rotterdam 2003	AE-PCOS society 2006
1. Irregular periods (≤8 menses/year 2. Elevated serum androgens/hyperandrogenemia 3. Polycystic ovarian morphology (ovarian volume >10 mL^3 or >12 follicles 2–9 mm in at least one ovary	1 and 2	Any 2 of 3	1 and 2 or 2 and 3

(NIH: National Institute of Health; AE: androgen excess; PCOS: polycystic ovary syndrome)

TABLE 2: PCOS phenotypes according to diagnostic criteria.

Phenotypes	1	2	3	4
	Classic	NIH	Ovulatory	Normoandrogenic
Hyperandrogenism	Yes	Yes	Yes	**No**
Chronic anovulation	Yes	Yes	**No**	Yes
Polycystic ovaries	Yes	**No**	Yes	Yes
NIH 1990	+	+	-	-
Rotterdam 2003	+	+	+	+
AE-PCOS society 2006	+	+	+	-

(NIH: National Institute of Health; AE: androgen excess; PCOS: polycystic ovary syndrome)

After exclusion of:

- Late onset *congenital adrenal hyperplasia* (CAH), androgen-secreting tumors, and Cushing's syndrome for elevated androgens
- Exclusion of thyroid disorders and elevated prolactin for oligo/anovulation
- Recent AE–PCOS society has recommended increase in the number of small follicles from >12 to ≥25.[2]

PATHOPHYSIOLOGY (FLOWCHART 1)

- *Genetics and PCOS*:
  - Regulatory gene of cytochrome P450 (CYP) 11A, FST, IVSR, 3–HSDL, and CYP enzyme[3]

Flowchart 1: Pathophysiology of polycystic ovarian syndrome (PCOS).

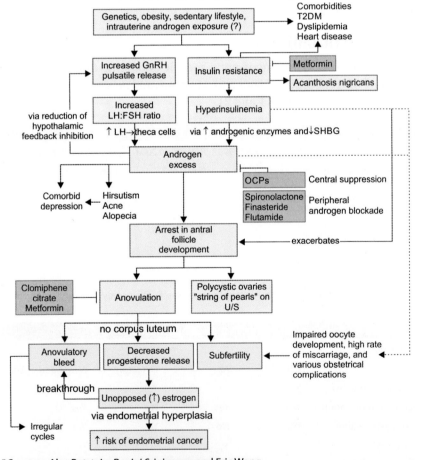

Courtesy: Alex Rotstein, Ragini Srinivasan, and Eric Wong.
(T2DM: type 2 diabetes mellitus; GnRH: gonadotropin releasing hormone; LH: luteinizing hormone; FSH: follicle stimulating hormone; OCPs: oral contraceptive pills; U/S: ultrasonography; SHBG: sex hormone binding globulin)

- – Theca cells are altered, with functional abnormality of 17- hydroxylase, which is rate limiting step in androgen biosynthesis[4]
- – Associated with disordered insulin metabolism and hyperinsulinemia **(Fig. 1)**[5]
- *Fetal origin of PCOS*:
  - – In utero programming is one of the postulated theories
  - – *Barker's hypothesis* (fetal origin of adult disease)
  - – In utero exposure to hyperandrogenemia → disturb epigenetic reprogramming
  - – In fetal reproductive system → PCOS phenotype after birth.

Fetal ovary and/or fetal adrenal are genetically predisposed to secrete excess androgens. The fetal ovary shows increased expression of P450c17 and androgen receptor during follicle formation **(Fig. 2)**.

■ CLINICAL FEATURES

- *Hyperandrogenism*: Acne (20–40%), *hirsutism* (75–80%), alopecia (less common).[6] The severity of *hirsutism* depends on the level of hyperandrogenemia, degree of adiposity, and genetic sensitivity of hair follicles to androgens.
- *Menstrual disturbances*: Seen in 60–85%.[7]

  It is seen as oligomenorrhea (47%), amenorrhea (51%), polymenorrhea (1.5–2.7%)[8]—normal cycles (12–20%), abnormal uterine bleeding (29%). Women with chronic anovulation, obesity, and hyperinsulinemia are at risk of developing endometrial cancer. So the decision for endometrial biopsy should be made based on the duration of exposure to unopposed estrogen stimulation, severity of obesity, and insulin resistance.

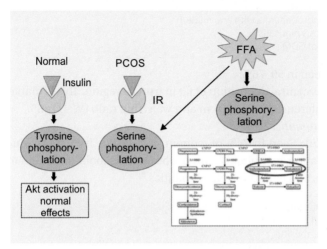

Fig. 1: Mechanism of IR in polycystic ovarian syndrome (PCOS).
(IR: insulin resistance; FFA: free fatty acids)

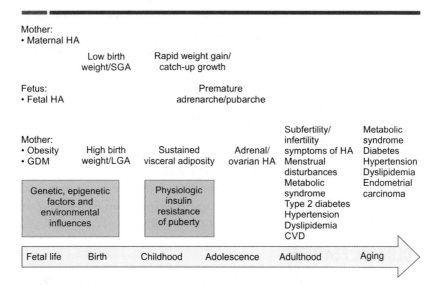

Fig. 2: Proposed evolution of PCOS from fetal life to adulthood.[6]
(CVD: cardiovascular disease; GDM: gestational diabetes; HA: hyperandrogenism; LGA: large for gestational age; SGA: small for gestational age)

ESHRE Capri Workshop Group Recommendation[8]

Screening strategy for PCOS
- Measure BMI and WC
- Lipid profile every 2 years if normal
- 2-hour GTT with 75 g glucose every 2 years if normal and earlier with risk factors. Consider using HbAiC
- Age > 40 years
- BMI > 25 kg/m² (Asian)
- W/H ratio > 0.85
- Hyperandrogenemia with anovulation
- Acanthosis nigricans
- History of GDM

Obesity: Seen in 50–76%.
- There is central deposition of fat in truncal region. This is marked by waist circumference (WC) ≥80 cm and waist/hip ratio (W/H) >85.
- *Asymptomatic:* 20%.
- *Infertility:* Seen in 74% of women with PCOS. It might be due to oligo/anovulation, combined factor of obesity, metabolic, inflammatory, oocyte quality, and endocrine abnormalities.[8]

Long-term sequel
- Impaired glucose tolerance
- Diabetes mellitus
- Cardiovascular disease

Contd...

Contd...

- Hypertension
- Dyslipidemia
- Nonalcoholic fatty liver disease
- Obstructive sleep apnea
- Psychological—anxiety, depression, behavioral disorders
- Endometrial carcinoma.

CLINICAL SIGNS

- *Acanthosis nigricans (Fig. 3)*:
  - Dark brown velvety thickened cutaneous plaques
  - On the back of the neck, axillae, beneath the breasts, elbows, and knuckles
  - Seen in 5–10% of PCOS and 50% of obese PCOS[8]
  - Secondary to insulin resistance with increased risk of diabetes mellitus, lipid dysfunction.
- *Hyperandrogenism:* Acne, *hirsutism*, alopecia.

ULTRASOUND FEATURES

- Polycystic ovarian morphology **(Fig. 4)**
  - Follicle number per ovary (FNPO) > 12, ov vol > 10 cc^3
  - Can be unilateral or bilateral
- AE–PCOS Society has recommended increase in the number of small follicles from >12 to ≥25[2]
- Stromal hyperechogenecity—due to increased stroma
- Peripheral distribution of antral follicles—"Necklace pattern"
- 3-D USG to assess:
  - Ovarian morphology
  - Ovarian stroma
  - Ovarian vascularization.

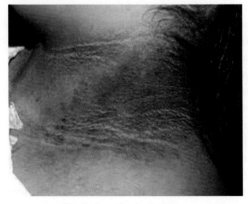

Fig. 3: Acanthosis nigricans.

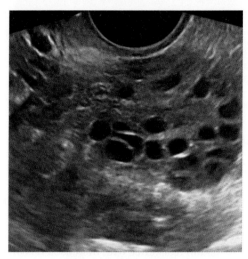

Fig. 4: Polycystic ovaries.

Evaluation of a women with suspected PCOS should include:
- Serum TSH, Prolactin
- 2-hour GTT with 75 g glucose
- Fasting lipid profile
- Serum testosterone
- Morning follicular phase 17-OH
- Progesterone (in pre or perimenarcheal onset of hirsutism)
- Family history of CAH, high risk ethnicity)
- 24-hour free cortisol - if suggestive of Cushing's syndrome.
- Overnight dexamethasone suppression test - if hypercortisolism is suspected.

MANAGEMENT

- It depends on the age, clinical manifestations, and concern for infertility.
- Treatment is a multidisciplinary approach involving gynecologist, pediatrician, endocrinologist, cardiologist, and geriatrician.
- *First-line treatment—Lifestyle modifications*
  - It includes weight loss in overweight and obese women.
    - *Weight loss*: 5–10% weight loss decreases testosterone levels, increase in sex hormone binding globulin (SHBG), decrease insulin resistance, and other metabolic derangements.
  - 30% reduction in visceral fat can normalize menstrual cycles in 44% of PCOS women and hence improves fertility.[9]
  - Low calorie diet of 1,000–1,200 kcal/day with low glycemic index and diet rich in fibers and high plant proteins. A calorie restriction of 500 kcal/day can reduce body weight by 10% in 6 months.[9]
    - *Exercise*: Aerobic exercise of 3–4 times/week for 20–30 minutes burn 100–200 kcal and 40% improvement in insulin sensitivity in 48 hours.[9] It is recommended to perform either 150 minutes of

moderate intensity exercise per week or 75 minutes of vigorous intensity exercise[10] and the latter reduce the risk of metabolic syndrome by 22%.[11]

- *Drugs*
  - Orlistat, a lipase inhibitor is tried in the dose of 120 mg thrice daily with meals. Other drugs approved by US-FDA are lorcaserin, phentermine with topiramate extended release, naltrexone sustained release, and liraglutide. As adverse effect profile is not clear, it is not widely used.[12]
- *Bariatric surgery*
  If BMI >40 kg/m^2 or 37 kg/m^2 if associated with metabolic syndrome.

Management of Hyperandrogenic Features

Hirsutism

Antiandrogens:
At least 6 months of therapy is required to see the therapeutic response.
- *Spironolactone*: 100–200 mg/day.
- *Flutamide*: 250 mg/day, less used due to dose dependent hepatotoxicity.
- *Finasteride*: 5 mg/day can cause feminization of male fetus, hence not used in reproductive age group.
- *Cyproterone acetate (CPA)*: Antiandrogen with progestogenic activity. It is given in the dose of 25–50 mg/day on cycle days 5–14 or along with ethinyl estradiol (EE) (CPA 2 mg+ EE 20 µg/day).
- Combined oral contraceptive pills (COC).
- COC with antiandrogenic progestins like CPA (2 mg), drospirenone (3 mg), and desogestrel (150 µg) are first-line agents when they are not planning to conceive.

Dermatological interventions:
- *Permanent methods*: Electrolysis and photoepilation devices (laser, intense pulse light).
- *Temporary methods*: Waxing, plucking, shaving, epilation, and bleaching.
- *Topical*: 1% eflornithine hydrochloride decrease unwanted facial hair growth.

Acne

- COC with CPA, drospirenone, desogestrel
- *Topical*: Salicylic acid, benzoyl peroxide, clindamycin/benzoyl peroxide, and tretinoin.

Alopecia

- *COC and androgen blockers*: First-line therapy.
- *Topical*: Minoxidil 2–5% twice daily.

Management of Menstrual Dysfunction

- *Combined oral contraceptive pills*: If not planning to conceive.
- This forms the first line of treatment for menstrual irregularity and hyperandrogenism.[7]
- The dose of EE varies from 20 to 35 µg and progestin with minimum androgenic property.
- *Progestin therapy*: When estrogen is contraindicated.
- Cyclical micronized progesterone (100–200 mg/day) or medroxyprogesterone acetate (10 mg/day) for 10–14 days a month.
- Other options to prevent endometrial hyperplasia: DMPA, LNG-IUS, *etonogestrel* implants.
- *Transdermal contraceptive patch* (0.75 mg EE + Norelgestromin 6 mg) is associated with increased risk of venous thromboembolism.[13]
- *Transvaginal contraceptive ring* (EE 15 µg + 120 µg *etonogestrel*/day over 3 weeks monthly.
- *RCOG guidelines*: In oligomenorrhea or *amenorrhea*, withdrawal bleeding should be induced every 3–4 months with cyclical progestogens for at least 12 days or COC or endometrial protection gained by exposure to gestogens by intrauterine device.[14]

Management of Infertility

Majority of patients have anovulation (74–80%).

Drugs for Ovulation Induction (OI)

- Selective estrogen receptor modulators **(SERMs)**
  - *Clomiphene citrate (CC)*
    - Drug of first choice for ovulation induction in women with anovulatory PCOS.
    - *Dose*: 50–150 mg/day from day 2/3 for 5 days.
    - Can also start with "stair step" protocol to reduce the number of cycles required for documenting ovulation.
    - *Outcome*: Ovulation rate—75–80%, conception rate/cycle—22–36%, multiple pregnancy rate (MPR)—8%, miscarriage rate—10–20%, live birth rate (LBR) after 6 cycles—20–29%.
    - *CC resistance*: It is defined as failure to ovulate after receiving CC 150 mg/day for 5 days per cycle for at least 3 cycles. This can occur in obese women insulin resistance and in hyperandrogenemia.
    - *In CC resistance, options available are*:
      - *Concomitant use of insulin sensitizers*: Metformin up to 1,500 g/day.
      - *Second-line therapy*: Gonadotropins/laparoscopic ovarian drilling

♦ Extended use of CC 100 mg/day for 7 or more days rarely up to 150 mg/day.

♦ Use of letrozole.

♦ *Addition of glucocorticoids*: Dexamethasone 0.25–0.5 mg or prednisolone 5 mg.

♦ Pretreatment with COC.

- *CC failure*: Those who ovulate but fail to conceive after three or more cycles of ovulation induction with CC and this warrants further evaluation.

– *Tamoxifen*:
  - SERM with estrogen antagonist action in breasts, peripheral sites and partial agonist action in uterus, bone, liver, and pituitary.
  - *Dose*: 20–40 mg/d from day 2/3 for 5 days.
  - Reasonably good results are seen in CC failure patients with beneficial effects on endometrium, cervix, bone mineral density, and serum lipids.[15]

Aromatase Inhibitors

- *Letrozole*:
  – Letrozole is commonly used aromatase inhibitors (AI) for ovulation induction.
  – However, recently letrozole has been considered as the first-line drug and gonadotropins as second-line drug. If these therapies have failed, then IVF can be offered.[7] ACOG has recommended letrozole as the first-line drug for ovulation induction in PCOS with BMI >30 kg/m^2 as there is increase in live birth.[16] The advantages of AI are: (1) No antiestrogenic action on endometrium and cervical mucus. (2) Short half-life of 45 hours leads to late follicular raise in estrogen with a shorter FSH window. This mimics the normal physiological cycle. (3) Promotes monofollicular development and hence decreased risk of ovarian hyperstimulation syndrome (OHSS) and multiple pregnancy.
  – *Outcomes*: Ovulation rate—75%, pregnancy rate (PR)—similar to CC
- *Anastrozole*:
  – It has been tried for OI
  – *Dose*: 1 mg/d from day 2/3 for 5 days.
- *Gonadotropins*:
  – They can be used alone or with oral ovulogens.
  – *Indications*:
    - Resistance or failure to CC/letrozole.
    - Persistent LH hypersecretion.
    - Cycles planned for intrauterine insemination (IUI).
    - In assisted reproductive technology (ART) cycles.

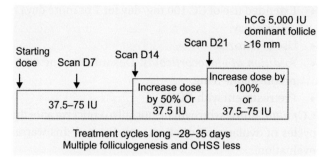

Fig. 5: Chronic low dose step up protocol.
(hCG: human chorionic gonadotropin; OHSS: ovarian hyperstimulation syndrome)

- Any of the gonadotropins [urine derived *follicle-stimulating hormone* (UFSH), highly purified follicle-stimulating hormone (hp-FSH), human menopausal gonadotropin (HMG), recombinant follicle stimulating hormone (rFSH)] can be used. There is no difference in pregnancy outcome and risk of OHSS.[17]
- Preferred stimulation protocols for IUI in PCOS women are chronic low dose step up protocol and low dose step up protocol **(Fig. 5)**.
- *Outcome*: PR: 20–25%/cycle, cumulative pregnancy rate: 50–70%, MPR: 10–30%, and OHSS: 2%.[10]
- Recommended guidelines for anovulatory CC resistant PCOS with no other factors for infertility, where gonadotropins are suitable for use, consideration should be to provide a low-dose protocol and appropriate monitoring to minimize the complications.[18]

Laparoscopic Ovarian Drilling (LOD)

- It is the laparoscopic creation of multiple punctures in the ovary through the capsule using electrocautery or laser. It can be second-line therapy if follicular monitoring is not feasible with gonadotropin treatment.
- *Indications*:
  - Anovulatory CC/letrozole resistance
  - Lean PCOS with serum LH >10 IU/L
  - Suitable in younger age women with duration of infertility <3 years, lean PCOS with elevated serum LH >10 IU/L and AMH ≤7.7 ng/mL with no associated causes for infertility.[19]
- It probably acts by destruction of androgen-producing stroma and thereby reduces the circulating androgen levels.
- *Advantages*:
  - Correction of hormonal milieu (↓ androgens, LH)
  - Monofolliculogenesis
  - Intensive monitoring not required
  - Reduced risk of multiple pregnancy, OHSS.

- *Disadvantages*:
  - Destruction of small follicles leads to drop in serum AMH levels and hence the ovarian reserve leads to premature ovarian insufficiency.
  - Periovarian adhesion formation—distort tubo-ovarian relationship.
- *Precautions to be taken*:
  - Avoid hilar region
  - Post-procedure wash with crystalloid solution
  - Avoid multiple punctures.
  - According to Cochrane review, there is no difference in MR, LBR, long-term cost, and *quality of life* (QoL). However, LOD was better than gonadotropins in reducing MPR and short-term cost.[20]

Assisted Reproductive Technology

- Anovulation per se is not an indication for ART.
- *Indications*:
  - Failure to conceive even after 6 cycles of OI with IUI.
  - *Coexistent factors*—advanced maternal age, tubal factor, male factor, need for PGT.
- GnRH antagonist protocol should be preferred as it is associated with shorter duration of stimulation, less dose of gonadotropins, can use agonist trigger and reduce risk of OHSS.
- CPR with fresh embryo transfer according to phenotypes are A (32.5%), B (26.4%), C (36.8%), and D (53.3%). This might be due to associated hyperandrogenism in A and B phenotypes.[21]

In Vitro Maturation (IVM)

- Immature oocytes are retrieved transvaginally and matured in vivo for 24–48 hours with FSH and hCG priming and then assessed for maturation. After denudation, ICSI is performed.
- This reduces the dose of gonadotropins, and avoids the risk of OHSS.
- When compared to IVF, CPR/cycle (45.8% vs. 32.4%) and LBR (40.7% vs. 23.5%) are lower with in vitro maturation (IVM).[22]
- In vitro maturation is yet to be adopted in routine clinical practice and still remains as a research entity.

Adjuvants in PCOS

Metformin

- It is shown to increase the ovulation rate in CC resistant PCOS, mediated partly by weight loss and reduction in androgen levels and insulin resistance. This also improves the folliculogenesis, embryo quality, and CPR.

- It is known to reduce the risk of moderate to severe OHSS if used for 12 weeks prior to ART by ameliorating the expression of VEGF.[23]
- Cochrane 2017 concluded that metformin may improve the menstrual frequency and ovulation rate and marginally improve the LBR. There is insufficient evidence to show the beneficial effect of metformin on multiple pregnancy and OHSS rates.[24]

Inositol-Myoinositol

At the level of ovary, it reduces hyperandrogenemia, regularizes menstrual cycle with spontaneous ovulation, improves the ovarian response, induces nuclear cytoplasmic maturation and hence the competence of the oocyte.[24,25]

D-chiro Inositol (DCI)

- Acts at the level of periphery—reduces IR, improves glucose metabolism, lipid profile, and hence reduces the cardiovascular and metabolic complications.[24]
- Better clinical results are ensured when MI and DCI are administered in the ratio of 40:1.[25]
- *Dose*: 2–4 g/day.

Vitamin D

- Even though its use is controversial, vitamin D supplementation has shown beneficial effects on IR, hyperandrogenism, follicular maturation, menstrual regularity, and ovulation.
- Vitamin D2 or D3 is given in the dose of 1,000–2,000 U/d or 50,000 U/week. It can be combined with calcium in the dose of 400 IU/d and 1,000 mg/day respectively for 3 months.

L-methylfolate

- It helps in DNA synthesis and reduces homocysteine levels thereby reducing the risk of cardiovascular risk factors.
- *Dose*: 1–5 mg/d for 3 months.

Antioxidants

N-acetyl cysteine
- It is a precursor of glutathione. Influence the insulin receptor activity and insulin secretion and hence increase the glucose utility.
- *Dose*: 600 mg twice daily for 6 weeks.
- Along with CC, it improves ovulation rate and pregnancy rate.

Melatonin
- It reduces intrafollicular oxidative damage, prevents DNA damage, reduces reactive oxygen species (ROS) hence improves follicular growth, maturation, ovulation, oocyte quality, and fertilization.
- Its use requires further clarity.

L-carnitine
- It reduces IR, improves lipid profile.
- It improves the ovulation rate and fertilization rate.
- *Dose*: 3 g/day for 8 weeks.

OCP pretreatment
- Suppress HPO axis, reduce LH and androgens, and improves folliculogenesis.
- But there is increase in the number of days of stimulation and the dose of gonadotropins.[26]
- *Statins* like simvastatin and atorvastatin are considered in the treatment of dyslipidemia. It is a category X drug, so should not be used when planning to conceive.
- **Glucagon-like peptide 1 receptor agonist** augments insulin secretion, inhibits glucagon secretion. It includes exenatide and liraglutide. Its combination with metformin for 12 weeks facilitates weight loss. However, larger studies are required.

POLYCYSTIC OVARY SYNDROME AND PREGNANCY

- Increased risk of:
  - Recurrent miscarriage (36–56%)
  - Gestational diabetes (40–50%)
  - Gestational hypertension (5%)
  - Neonatal complications—SGA (10–155) NICU admissions.
- These complications are more in phenotype A and B, due to impaired early decidual trophoblastic invasion.

POLYCYSTIC OVARY SYNDROME AND MENOPAUSE

- Increased risk of endometrial hyperplasia and endometrial carcinoma (3 fold)
- Increased risk of cardiovascular event.

ADOLESCENT POLYCYSTIC OVARY SYNDROME (FLOWCHARTS 2 AND 3)

- For diagnosis of adolescent PCOS, all three components—hyperandrogenism, ovulatory dysfunction, and PCO morphology must be present as per Rotterdam criteria.[9,10]

Flowchart 2: Irregular cycles, amenorrhea, and ovulatory dysfunction in adolescents.

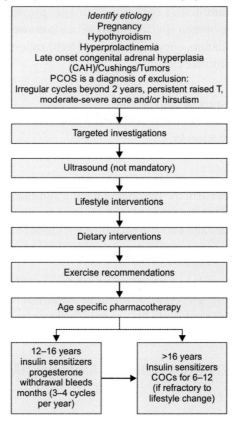

- Accepted *diagnostic factors* and pathognomonic markers include:[27]
  - Early acne or hirsutism; persistent hirsutism
  - Persistent severe acne; frequent relapse in acne
  - Acanthosis nigricans
  - Alopecia
  - Family history in sibling and mother
  - Obesity and inadequate lifestyle
  - Markers of lipid dysregulation
- *Targeted investigations* should include:

Urine pregnancy test	Pregnancy
FSH-LH	Hypo/hypergonadism
Prolactin assessment	Hyperprolactinemia
Thyroid function tests	Hypothyroidism
17-OH-progesterone	Late onset CAH
Lipid profile	Early metabolic syndrome

Flowchart 3: Obesity in adolescents.

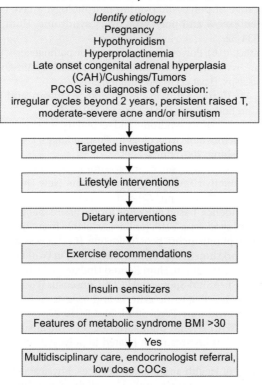

Identify etiology
Pregnancy
Hypothyroidism
Hyperprolactinemia
Late onset congenital adrenal hyperplasia
(CAH)/Cushings/Tumors
PCOS is a diagnosis of exclusion:
irregular cycles beyond 2 years, persistent raised T,
moderate-severe acne and/or hirsutism

↓

Targeted investigations

↓

Lifestyle interventions

↓

Dietary interventions

↓

Exercise recommendations

↓

Insulin sensitizers

↓

Features of metabolic syndrome BMI >30

↓ Yes

Multidisciplinary care, endocrinologist referral,
low dose COCs

- **Role of ultrasound[7]**
  - Ultrasound should not be used for the diagnosis of PCOS in those with gynecological age of <8 years (<8 years after menarche), due to the high incidence of multi-follicular ovaries in this life stage.
  - The transvaginal ultrasound approach is preferred in the diagnosis of PCOS, if sexually active and if acceptable to the individual being assessed.
  - Using endovaginal ultrasound transducers, the threshold for PCOM should be in either ovary, a follicle number per ovary of >20 and/or an ovarian volume ≥10 mL, ensuring no corpora luteal cysts or dominant follicles are present. In transabdominal ultrasound in adolescents, reporting is best focused on ovarian volume with a threshold of ≥12 mL for both ovaries or a single ovary ≥ 15 mL, given the difficulty of reliably assessing follicle number with this approach.[27]

■ REFERENCES

1. Johnstone EB, Rosen MP, Neril R, Trevithick D, Sternfeld B, Murphy R, et al. The polycystic ovary post–Rotterdam: a common, age-dependent finding in ovulatory women without metabolic significance. J Clin Endocrinol Metab. 2010;95(11): 4965-72.

2. Dewally D, Lijan ME, Carmina E, Cedars MI, Laven J, Norman RJ, et al. Definition and significance of polycystic ovarian morphology: a task force report from the androgen excess and polycystic ovary syndrome. Hum Reprod Update. 2014;20(3):334-52.
3. Yolanda Smith. (2016). Polycystic ovary syndrome pathogenesis. [online] Available from: https://www.news-medical.net/health/Polycystic-Ovary-Syndrome-Pathogenesis.aspx. [Last accessed January, 2020].
4. Barber TM, Mc Carthy MI, Wass JA, Franks S. Obesity and polycystic ovary syndrome. Clin Endocrinol (Oxf). 2006; 65(2):137-45.
5. Balen AH. Polycystic ovary syndrome and secondary amenorrhoea. In: Dewhurst's Textbook of Obstetrics and Gynecology for Postgraduates, 17th edition. New Jersey: Black well publishing; 2007. pp. 377-98.
6. Krishna D, Rao KA. Polycystic ovary syndrome. In: Principles and Practice of Assisted Reproductive Technology, 2nd edition. New Delhi: Jaypee Brothers Medical Publishers (P) Ltd. pp. 479–521.
7. International evidence-based guideline for the assessment and management of polycystic ovary syndrome 2018. [online] Available from: https://www.monash.edu/medicine/sphpm/mchri/pcos/guideline. [Last accessed January, 2020]
8. ESHRE Capri Workshop Group. Health and fertility in World Health Organization group 2 anovulatory women. Hum Reprod Update. 2012:18(5):586-99.
9. Rotterdam ESHRE/ASRM-Sponsored PCOS Consensus Workshop Group. Revised 2003 consensus on diagnostic criteria and long-term health risks related to polycystic ovary syndrome. Fertil Steril. 2004;81:19-25.
10. Thessaloniki ESHRE/ASRM-Sponsored PCOS Consensus Workshop Group. Consensus on infertility treatment related to polycystic ovary syndrome. Hum Reprod 2008;23:462-77.
11. US Department of Health and Human Services. Physical activity and health: A report of the surgeon general. [online] Available from: https://www.cdc.gov/nccdphp/sgr/pdf/sgrfull.pdf. [Last accessed January, 2020].
12. Derosa G, Maffioli P. Anti-obesity drugs: a review about their effects and their safety. Expert Opin Drug Saf. 2012;11(3):459-71.
13. Diamanti-Kandarakis E. Polycystic ovarian syndrome: pathophysiology, molecular aspects and clinical implications. Expert Rev Mol Med. 2008;10:e3.
14. Royal college of Obstetricians and Gynecologist. (2014) Long-term consequences of Polycystic ovary syndrome. Green-top Guideline No. 33. [online] Available from: https://www.rcog.org.uk/globalassets/documents/guidelines/gtg_33.pdf. [Last accessed January, 2020].
15. Steiner AZ1, Terplan M, Paulson RJ. Comparison of tamoxifen and clomiphene citrate for ovulation induction: a meta-analysis. Hum Reprod. 2005;20(6):1511-5.
16. American College of Obstetrician and Gynecologist. (2018). Aromatase Inhibitors in Gynecologic Practice; A committee opinion, Number 738. [online] Available from: https://www.acog.org/-/media/Committee-Opinions/Committee-on-Gynecologic-Practice/co738.pdf?dmc=1&ts=20200102T1241486461. [Last accessed January, 2020].
17. Weiss NS, Nahuis M, Mol BWJ, van der Veen F, van Wely M. Gonadotrophins for ovulation induction in women with polycystic ovarian syndrome. Cochrane Systematic Review. 2015;(9):CD010290.
18. Balen AH, Morley LC, Misso M, Franks S, Legro RS, Wijeyaratne CN, et al. The management of anovulatory infertility in women with polycystic ovary syndrome: an analysis of the evidence to support the development of global WHO guidance. Hum Reprod Update. 2016;22(6):687-708.

19. Amer SAK, Li TC, Ledger WL. Ovulation induction using laparoscopic ovarian drilling in women with polycystic ovarian syndrome: predictors of success. Hum Reprod. 2004;19(8):1719-24.

20. Farquhar C, Brown J, Marjoribanks J. Laparoscopic drilling by diathermy or laser for ovulation induction in anovulatory polycystic ovary syndrome. Cochrane Database Syst Rev. 2012;(6):CD001122.

21. Ramezanali F, Ashrafi M, Hemat M, Arabipoor A, Jalali S, Moini A. Assisted reproductive outcomes in women with different polycystic ovary syndrome phenotypes: the predictive value of anti-Müllerian hormone. Reprod Biomed Online. 2016;32(5):503-12.

22. Siristatidis CS, Vrachnis N, Creatsa M, Maheshwari A, Bhattacharya S. In vitro maturation in subfertile women with polycystic ovarian syndrome undergoing assisted reproduction. Cochrane Database Syst Rev. 2013; (10):CD 006606.

23. Tso LO, Costello MF, Albuquerque LE, Andriolo RB, Freitas V. Metformin treatment before and during IVF or ICSI in women with polycystic ovary syndrome. Cochrane Database Syst Rev. 2009;(2):CD 006105.

24. Unfer V, Carlomagno G, Dante G, Facchinetti F. Effects of myo-inositol in women with PCOS: a meta-analysis of randomized controlled trials. Gynecol Endocrinol. 2012;28(7):509-15.

25. Tang T, Lord JM, Norman RJ, Yasmin E, Balen AH. Insulin-sensitising drugs (metformin, rosiglitazone, pioglitazone, D-chiro-inositol) for women with polycystic ovary syndrome, oligo amenorrhoea and subfertility. Cochrane Database Syst Rev. 2012;(5):CD003053.

26. Griesinger G, Venetis CA, Marx T, Diedrich K, Tarlatzis BC, Kolibianakis EM. Oral contraceptive pill pretreatment in ovarian stimulation with GnRH antagonists for IVF: a systematic review and meta-analysis. Fertil Steril. 2008;90(4):1055-63.

27. Malik S, Jain K, Talwar P, Prasad S, Dhorepatil B, Devi G, et al. Management of polycystic ovary syndrome in India. Fertility Science & Research. 2014;1(1):23-4.

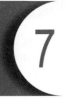

7

Current Concepts in Ovulation Induction

Nandita Palshetkar, Rohan Palshetkar, Jiteeka Thakkar

BACKGROUND

Anovulatory infertility is a common problem faced in infertility practice. The causes of anovulation have been classified by the World Health Organization into three categories based on the gonadotropin profile:

WHO type 1 (hypogonadotropic hypogonadism) (10%): It is caused by any lesion affecting the pituitary or hypothalamus and affecting gonadotropin production including idiopathic, weight-related amenorrhea, Sheehan syndrome, extreme stress and strenuous exercise, Kallmann syndrome, craniopharyngiomas, etc.

WHO type 2 (normogonadotropic hypogonadism): The most common cause of anovulation accounting for 85% of cases and is most commonly caused by polycystic ovarian syndrome. Hyperprolactinemic amenorrhea is another cause, where in addition to amenorrhea and infertility, women may have galactorrhea.

WHO type 3 (hypergonadotropic hypogonadism) (5%): This is usually an indication of ovarian failure.

TREATMENT STRATEGIES AND GOALS

In anovulatory women, the purpose of treatment in ovulation induction is the development of at least one follicle, whereas in other causes of infertility, ovarian stimulation is used to increase the number of follicles, known as super ovulation or controlled ovarian hyperstimulation. Induction of ovulation is possible in the first two types. However, in the third type, ovulation induction is usually unsuccessful due to follicular depletion and the only way to achieve a pregnancy may be through oocyte donation.

CLOMIPHENE CITRATE

Clomiphene is being used for over five decades for ovulation induction. It is similar in structure to estrogen and thus binding to estrogen receptors.[1] While most modern fertility physicians have now shifted to aromatase inhibitors (AIs) as a first-line agent for oral ovulation induction, the role of clomiphene citrate (CC) and the significant body of evidence on this molecule built up over several decades needs to be discussed.

As a selective estrogen receptor modulator (SERM), clomiphene acts both as an agonist as well as an antagonist. For ovulation induction, the agonist feature of CC is most vital to us.[2] Clomiphene binds to estrogen receptors and provides a false sensation of low estrogen state to the hypothalamus. This causes the hypothalamic-pituitary-ovarian (HPO) axis to increase gonadotropin-releasing hormone (GnRH) secretion which in turn increases the release of gonadotropins.[1]

Treatment Regimen

Clomiphene citrate is generally started from day 2 to day 5 after the onset of menses. The rate of ovulation and pregnancy is similar irrespective of the day of menses on which clomiphene is started. Treatment with CC is associated with higher rate of pregnancy if started early (days 1 through 5 than 5 through 9) in the menstrual cycle.[3] Ideally, clomiphene is started at a dose of 50 mg/ day for 5 days. Ovulation generally occurs 5–10 days after the last CC dose. If a patient remains anovulation then the dose should be increased by 50 mg/day. Generally, a patient should ovulate with a dose of 50–150 mg/day.

In women who ovulate, 52% do so taking 50 mg, 22% taking 100 mg, and fewer with subsequent increases.[4] FDA does not approve a dose more than 100 mg/day while the American College of Obstetrics and Gynecology gives approval for dose up to 150 mg/day. This higher dose is generally required for women with slightly higher body mass index (BMI).[5]

Indications

Anovulatory Infertility

Traditionally, clomiphene has been the first-line treatment for anovulatory and oligo-ovulatory women, though recent guidance has now advocated the use of AIs as the first line of therapy, especially in polycystic ovary syndrome (PCOS) as per the new American Society for Reproductive Medicine/European Society of Human Reproduction and Embryology (ASRM/ESHRE) joint PCOS Guideline.[6]

Unexplained Infertility

In unexplained infertility, clomiphene is used rampantly. However, there is no evidence which supports significant benefit over a placebo in planned relations cycle. Clomiphene citrate when combined with intrauterine insemination (IUI) has shown benefit over a placebo.[7]

Clomiphene citrate is an efficient, inexpensive, and well-tolerated drug with a well-known safety profile when used correctly.[8] A recent review supports the use of CC as first-line treatment for ovulation induction in PCOS.[9] The continuation of treatment for another six cycles of CC before switching to, for example, gonadotropins may be cost-effective theoretically.[9,10]

TAMOXIFEN

Tamoxifen is another SERM which is similar to CC and has proven successfully as an ovulation induction agent.[11] Traditionally, it has been used in the medical management of breast cancer. However, the lack of data and prevalence of side effect such as hot flashes have limited its use in clinical practice.

Aromatase Inhibitors

Aromatase inhibitors such anastrozole and letrozole have been used for ovulation inductions.[12] They prevent aromatization and this prevents androgens from being converted to estrogen. This causes a low estrogenic state. And therefore acts on HPO axis and pituitary. This causes compensatory increase in the pulsatile GnRH secretion and thereby causes follicular growth.[2]

Post letrozole supplementation, estrogen levels increase immediately, which causes an abrupt decrease in follicle-stimulating hormone (FSH) levels. This ensures monofollicular growth and the increase in estrogen helps in endometrial preparation and production of cervical mucus.

Therapy Regimen and Efficacy

Letrozole doses can be started from 2.5 mg/day to 7.5 mg/day. Anastrozole is given as 1 mg daily. Both medications are started as per the CC protocol. Extended regimens (10 days) and single dose regimens (20 mg on day 3), have also been used with studies suggesting positive results.[13,14]

Letrozole can be combined with planned relations or IUI. In anovulatory women, AIs have shown almost a 60% ovulation rate with pregnancy rates varying from 12% to 40%.[15,16]

Indications

Letrozole is indicated in women who are resistant to CC or those women in which CC is contraindicated due to undesirable side effects.[17] Aromatase inhibitor can also be implemented in cases where the endometrium is thin (<7 mm) where CC was used as oral ovulogen.[18,19]

In a recent Cochrane review, PCOS patients seem to have better pregnancy as well as live birth rate when letrozole was used.[20] This differs from a previous review, which did not detect a difference.[21]

ADJUVANT REGIMENS

These have traditionally been described in textbooks of reproductive endocrinology (especially glucocorticoids and bromocriptine) and are mentioned here for completeness; their utility is restricted in day-to-day practice.

Clomiphene and Glucocorticoids

With normal and elevated levels of dehydroepiandrosterone (DHEA) in CC-resistant patients, addition of dexamethasone (0.5–2 mg) or prednisolone (5 mg) has shown increase in ovulation and pregnancy rates. The mechanism of action is not clearly known but there is a hypothesis that suggests the androgen suppression has direct effects on the oocyte and indirect effects on cytokines and intrafollicular growth factors.[16]

Clomiphene and Human Chorionic Gonadotropin

Human chorionic gonadotropin (hCG) injection may benefit as surrogate luteinizing hormone (LH) surge to trigger ovulation in patients where CC is used especially in cases of unexplained infertility or coexisting male factor.

Clomiphene and Metformin

Metformin should be considered in combination with CC in patients who are CC resistant. Metformin is usually given in a dose of 1,500–2,000 mg/day. The starting dose of 500 mg/day should be given after which the dose should be increased to the require dose. A liver function test should always be carried out prior to starting metformin.

A meta-analysis has suggested that metformin may improve success in weight management.[22] Otherwise, the role of metformin in ovulation induction is controversial. Interestingly, metformin may have a role as pretreatment before standard assisted reproduction techniques. A recent randomized controlled trial (RCT) demonstrated improved pregnancy rates after 3–9 months of metformin before assisted reproduction techniques.[23]

Exogenous Gonadotropins

Gonadotropins were first obtained by purifying urine; nowadays many commercially available preparations are from highly purified urinary source medications or are the product of recombinant technology. The major boon of recombinant gonadotropins is that they provide a more consistent supply, there is barely any variation in the activity of the molecule and the biggest advantage is that there is antigenic urinary protein present.[2,24]

Indications

Hypogonadotropic Hypogonadism

In WHO group 1 patients, oral ovulogens are generally not effective, especially those patients who do not have an intact HPO axis. In such patients, exogenous FSH and LH restore ovulation in these patients.[25]

Clomiphene Citrate Resistant Anovulation

The WHO group 2 patients who do not respond to oral ovulogens should be subjected to exogenous FSH and LH. Exogenous gonadotropins should be used as second line of treatment for ovulation induction.[6]

Unexplained Infertility

Superovulation is often the goal of using gonadotropins in this population attempting to optimize cycle fecundity.

Therapy Regimen and Efficacy

As a prerequisite, extensive counseling is essential. The couple must understand the expected expenditure and time that needs to be committed for monitoring the effects of the medicine. Serum estradiol levels as well as follicular number and growth must be monitored to prevent ovarian hyperstimulation syndrome (OHSS). The dose and duration of gonadotropins depends on age, BMI, and ovarian reserve of the patients.

The *"step-up"* protocol is aimed at crossing the FSH threshold and reduces the risk of complications. The drawback of this protocol is that increases the duration of the cycle and can result in multifollicular growth.

The *"step-down"* protocol overcomes these problems by replicating the hormonal cycle. Follicle-stimulating hormone (FSH) is started at a higher dose so that the dominant follicle develops faster. Once the dominant follicle is established, the FSH levels can be reduced slowly to ensure monofollicular growth.[10]

It is important to monitor the patients, because the FSH window needs to be managed to ensure either mono- or multifollicular growth. The cycle can be cancelled if there are more than three dominant follicles. The biggest concern of the step down protocol is starting the patient with a high initial dose of FSH whose threshold is low.

A low dose or chronic low dose step-up regimen may be considered in the first cycle to gauge a response for an individual patient. Eventually, the other cycles can be done depending on the response in the first cycle.

GnRH Agonists and Antagonists

Among the various GnRH agonist protocols, namely ultrashort, short and long, the long GnRH agonist protocol has been used as the gold standard in in vitro fertilization (IVF) since its discovery in the 1980s. GnRH antagonists have recently offered an alternative approach in IVF treatment.

The long GnRH agonist protocol involves administration of 0.1 mg GnRH agonist (e.g., triptorelin/leuprolide) starting on preceding cycle-day 21 followed by administration of gonadotropin at 150–225 IU (International Units) daily starting on cycle-day 2. The adjustment of dose is based on follicular development and administration of GnRH agonist and gonadotropin lasts until the hCG trigger injection, which is around 14 days post GnRH agonist regimen or when follicles reach 16–18 mm in size.

For the GnRH antagonist protocol, administration of gonadotropin is initiated after monitoring of patients' follicles sizes on cycle-day 2/3. Gonadotropin dosage varies according to the follicular response. Approximately after the 6th day of gonadotropin injection or when follicular size reaches ≥14 mm, subcutaneous administration of the GnRH antagonist (e.g., cetrorelix 0.25 mg/day) begins.

Myoinositol

It has been found in recent studies that insulin sensitizers like myoinositol improved the ovulation and pregnancy rate in insulin-resistant patients with PCOS when given alone or in combination with CC.[26]

J Pundir et al. conducted a systematic review and meta-analysis on inositol treatment in women with polycystic ovarian syndrome, published in the BJOG in 2017. 10 trials and a total of 362 women were on inositol (257 on myoinositol; 105 on di-chiro-inositol), 179 were on placebo, and 60 were on metformin. Inositol was associated with significantly improved ovulation rate [risk ratio (RR) 2.3; 95% confidence interval (CI) 1.1–4.7; I2 = 75%] and increased frequency of menstrual cycles (RR 6.8; 95% CI 2.8–16.6; I2 = 0%) compared with placebo. One study reported on clinical pregnancy rate with inositol compared with placebo (RR 3.3; 95% CI 0.4–27.1), and one study compared with metformin (RR 1.5; 95% CI 0.7–3.1). No studies evaluated live birth and miscarriage rates.[27]

They concluded that inositol appears to regulate menstrual cycles, improve ovulation, and induce metabolic changes in PCOS; however, evidence is lacking for pregnancy, miscarriage or live birth. A further, well-designed multicentric trial to address this issue to provide robust evidence of benefit is warranted.

■ COCHRANE META-ANALYSIS

Forty-two RCTs and 7,935 women were analyzed in a Cochrane meta-analysis in 2018.[20] Letrozole had higher live birth rates compared to clomiphene (with timed intercourse) [odds ratio (OR) 1.68, 95% CI 1.42–1.99; 2,954 participants; 13 studies; I2 = 0%; number needed to treat for an additional beneficial outcome (NNTB) = 10].

There is evidence for a higher pregnancy rate in favor of letrozole (OR 1.56, 95% CI 1.37 to 1.78; 4,629 participants; 25 studies; I2 = 1%; NNTB = 10; moderate-quality evidence). There is little or no difference between treatment groups in the rate of miscarriage by pregnancy (20% with CC vs. 19% with letrozole; OR 0.94, 95% CI 0.70–1.26; 1,210 participants; 18 studies; I2 = 0%) and multiple pregnancy rate (1.7% with CC vs. 1.3% with letrozole; OR 0.69, 95% CI 0.41 to 1.16; 3,579 participants; 17 studies; I2 = 0%).

There is low-quality evidence that live birth rates are similar with letrozole or laparoscopic ovarian drilling (OR 1.38, 95% CI 0.95–2.02; 548 participants; 3 studies; I2 = 23%). There is low-quality evidence that pregnancy rates are similar (OR 1.28, 95% CI 0.94–1.74; 774 participants; 5 studies; I2 = 0%). There is insufficient evidence for a difference in miscarriage rate (OR 0.66, 95% CI 0.30–1.43; 240 participants; 5 studies; I2 = 0%), or multiple pregnancies (OR 3.00, 95% CI 0.12–74.90; 548 participants; 3 studies; I2 = 0%).

Additional comparisons were made for letrozole versus placebo, SERMs followed by IUI, FSH, anastrozole, as well as dosage and administration protocols. There is insufficient evidence for a difference in either group of treatment due to a limited number of studies. Hence, the reviewers concluded that more research is necessary.[20]

CONCLUSION

Although CC as a treatment modality has existed for more than 50 years, an increased awareness of the effect of obesity and different PCOS phenotypes has emerged. Accordingly, ovulation induction in women suffering from oligo- and anovulation seeking fertility treatment has to be individualized according to weight, treatment efficacy, and patient compliance, with the aim of achieving monofollicular growth, mono-ovulation, and subsequently the birth of a singleton baby.

REFERENCES

1. Practice Committee of the American Society for Reproductive Medicine. Use of clomiphene citrate in infertile women: a committee opinion. Fertil Steril. 2013;100(2):341-8.
2. Fritz MA, Speroff L. Clinical Gynecologic Endocrinology and Infertility, 8th edition. Philadelphia: Wolters Kluwer Health/Lippincott Williams & Wilkins; 2011. p. 1439.
3. Dehbashi S, Vafaei H, Parsanezhad MD, Alborzi S. Time of initiation of clomiphene citrate and pregnancy rate in polycystic ovarian syndrome. Int J Gynaecol Obstet. 2006;93(1):44-8.
4. Von Hofe J, Bates GW. Ovulation induction. Obstet Gynecol Clin North Am. 2015;42:27-37.
5. American College of Obstetricians and Gynecologists. ACOG practice bulletin. Management of infertility caused by ovulatory dysfunction. Number 34, February 2002. American College of Obstetricians and Gynecologists. Int J Gynaecol Obstet. 2002;77(2):177-88.
6. Thessaloniki ESHRE/ASRM-Sponsored PCOS Consensus Workshop Group. Consensus on infertility treatment related to polycystic ovary syndrome. Fertil Steril. 2008;89(3):505-22.
7. Deaton JL, Gibson M, Blackmer KM, Nakajima ST, Badger GJ, Brumsted JR. A randomized, controlled trial of clomiphene citrate and intrauterine insemination in couples with unexplained infertility or surgically corrected endometriosis. Fertil Steril. 1990;54(6):1083-8.
8. Birch Petersen K, Pedersen NG, Pedersen AT, Lauritsen MP, la Cour Freiesleben N. Mono-ovulation in women with polycystic ovary syndrome: a clinical review on ovulation induction. Reprod Biomed Online. 2016;32(6):563-83.

9. Moolenaar LM, Nahuis MJ, Hompes PG, van der Veen F, Mol BW. Cost-effectiveness of treatment strategies in women with PCOS who do not conceive after six cycles of clomiphene citrate. Reprod Biomed Online. 2014;28:606-13.

10. van Santbrink EJ, Donderwinkel PF, van Dessel TJ, Fauser BC. Gonadotropin induction of ovulation using a step-down dose regimen: single-centre clinical experience in 82 patients. Hum Reprod. 1995;10:1048-53.

11. Dhaliwal LK, Suri V, Gupta KR, Sahdev S. Tamoxifen: an alternative to clomiphene in women with polycystic ovary syndrome. J Hum Reprod Sci. 2011;4(2):76-9.

12. Palomba S. Aromatase inhibitors for ovulation induction. J Clin Endocrinol Metab. 2015;100:1742-7.

13. Mitwally MF, Casper RF. Single-dose administration of an aromatase inhibitor for ovarian stimulation. Fertil Steril. 2005;83(1):229-31.

14. Atay V, Cam C, Muhcu M, Cam M, Karateke A. Comparison of letrozole and clomiphene citrate in women with polycystic ovaries undergoing ovarian stimulation. J Int Med Res. 2006;34(1):73-6.

15. Badawy A, Mosbah A, Tharwat A, Eid M. Extended letrozole therapy for ovulation induction in clomiphene-resistant women with polycystic ovary syndrome: a novel protocol. Fertil Steril. 2009;92(1):236-9.

16. Keay SD, Jenkins JM. Adjunctive use of dexamethasone in Clomid resistant patients. Fertil Steril 2003;80(1):230-1 [author reply: 231].

17. Nahid L, Sirous K. Comparison of the effects of letrozole and clomiphene citrate for ovulation induction in infertile women with polycystic ovary syndrome. Minerva Ginecol. 2012;64(3):253-8.

18. Mitwally MF, Casper RF. Use of an aromatase inhibitor for induction of ovulation in patients with an inadequate response to clomiphene citrate. Fertil Steril. 2001;75(2):305-9.

19. Begum MR, Ferdous J, Begum A, Quadir E. Comparison of efficacy of aromatase inhibitor and clomiphene citrate in induction of ovulation in polycystic ovarian syndrome. Fertil Steril. 2009;92(3):853-7.

20. Franik S, Eltrop SM, Kremer JAM, Kiesel L, Farquhar C. Aromatase inhibitors (letrozole) for subfertile women with polycystic ovary syndrome. Cochrane Database Syst Rev. 2018;5:CD010287.

21. Misso ML1, Wong JL, Teede HJ. Aromatase inhibitors for PCOS: a systematic review and meta-analysis. Hum Reprod Update. 2012;18(3):301-12.

22. Naderpoor N, Shorakae S, de Courten B, Misso ML, Moran LJ, Teede HJ. Metformin and lifestyle modification in polycystic ovary syndrome: systematic review and meta-analysis. Hum Reprod Update. 2015;21:560-74.

23. Morin-Papunen L, Rantala AS, Unkila-Kallio L, Tiitinen A, Hippelainen M, Perheentupa A, et al. Metformin improves pregnancy and live-birth rates in women with polycystic ovary syndrome (PCOS): a multicenter, double-blind, placebo-controlled randomized trial. J Clin Endocrinol Metab. 2012;97:1492-500.

24. Lathi RB, Milki AA. Recombinant gonadotropins. Curr Womens Health Rep. 2001;1(2):157-63.

25. Agents stimulating gonadal function in the human. Report of a WHO scientific group. World Health Organ Tech Rep Ser. 1973;514:1-30.

26. Kamenov Z, Kolarov G, Gateva A, Carlomagno G, Genazzani AD. Ovulation induction with myo-inositol alone and in combination with clomiphene citrate in polycystic ovarian syndrome patients with insulin resistance. Gynecol Endocrinol. 2015;31(2):131-5.

27. Pundir J, Psaroudakis D, Savnur P, Bhide P, Sabatini L, Teede H, et al. Inositol treatment of anovulation in women with polycystic ovary syndrome: a meta-analysis of randomised trials. BJOG. 2017;125(3):299-308.

8

Preimplantation Genetic Testing

Hrishikesh Pai, Rushika Mistry

■ BACKGROUND

In vitro fertilization (IVF) has revolutionized the treatment of infertility and is estimated to have led to more than 6 million births all over the world. It is now possible to test embryos formed by IVF for genetic diseases by utilizing preimplantation genetic testing (PGT). The primary goal of PGT is to identify genetic defects in embryos created through IVF before transferring them to the uterus, thus decreasing abortions and births with genetic abnormalities.

■ DEFINITIONS

The terms preimplantation genetic screening (PGS) and preimplantation genetic diagnosis (PGD) are now replaced by new terminology in the international glossary of infertility and fertility care.

PGT-A: Preimplantation Genetic Testing for Aneuploidy

This is routine screening of embryos to identify euploid embryos for transfer and screen and exclude those embryos with sporadic chromosome abnormality. It is therefore used to select embryos that are most likely to result in a successful pregnancy.

PGT-M: Preimplantation Genetic Testing for Monogenic/Single Gene Disorders

This is typically used when parents are known carriers of a single gene mutation. It is used to help reduce the risk to have a child with a known inherited disorder caused by a single gene.

PGT-SR: Preimplantation Genetic Testing for Structural Rearrangement

Commonly used when one of the parents is a known carrier of a balanced or Robertsonian translocation (structural chromosomal rearrangement). The resulting embryos may carry imbalance in chromosome number indicative of translocation. It reduces the risk of having a pregnancy or a child with an unbalanced structural abnormality.

■ INDICATIONS

- Advanced maternal age
- Recurrent pregnancy loss
- Multiple IVF failures
- Male factor infertility
- Patients with a family history of X-linked disorders with 25% risk of having an affected embryo
- Carriers of autosomal recessive disease
- Carriers of autosomal dominant diseases
- Human leukocyte antigen (HLA) matching.

■ GENETIC ABNORMALITIES THAT CAN BE DETECTED USING PGT

Aneuploidy

This is the presence of an abnormal number of chromosomes in a cell, instead of the usual 46 chromosomes. It does not include a difference of one or more complete sets of chromosomes.

Trisomy

It is a type of polysomy in which there are three instances of a particular chromosome, instead of the normal two. A trisomy is a type of aneuploidy.

Tetrasomy

It is a form of aneuploidy with the presence of four copies, instead of the normal two, of a particular chromosome.

Monosomy

It is a condition of having a diploid chromosome complement in which one chromosome lacks its homologous partner.

Nullisomy

It is a genome mutation where a pair of homologous chromosomes, that would normally be present, is missing.

Single Gene Disorder

Single gene disorder, also known as monogenic disease, is when a single mutation in a specific gene leads to a hereditary disease, which can occur early during childhood or have a late onset.

Mosaicism

The presence of two or more different cells lines with different chromosomal number or structure in one embryo resulted by errors in chromosomal segregation during mitosis. Mosaicism could be present only in the intermediate cell mass (ICM) and not in the trophectoderm (TE). It may be misdiagnosed as a euploid embryo and could result in an unfavorable outcome. It is advisable to perform amniocentesis/chorionic villus sampling (CVS) for confirmation of test results.

MitoScore: Mitochondria play an important role in energy production and have their own DNA that is known as mitochondrial DNA or mtDNA, which is responsible for predicting implantation potential of embryo. The mitochondrial score "MitoScore" represents the total mtDNA content in euploid embryos.

■ GENETIC ANALYSIS TECHNIQUES AVAILABLE FOR TESTING

There are three main techniques available for testing and are as described here.

Fluorescence In Situ Hybridization

Fluorescence in situ hybridization (FISH) is a molecular cytogenetic technique that uses fluorescent probes that bind to only those parts of a nucleic acid sequence with a high degree of complementarity of sequence.[1] Fluorescence microscopy can be used to find out where the fluorescent probe is bound to the chromosome.

It analyzes a limited number of chromosomes at a time (13, 16, 18, 21, 22, X, and Y). It was the initial method used for analysis because of its accuracy in results, but it has its technical limitations like the number of probes required to get reliable reports and the requirement of specific parent karyotyping prior to testing.

Array Comparative Genomic Hybridization

Array comparative genomic hybridization (CGH) is a molecular cytogenetic technique for the detection of chromosomal copy number changes on a genome with a high resolution scale. It is a significant advance in technology that allows detection of chromosome imbalances that are too small to be detected by microscope. It allows locus by locus measure of CNV (copy number variation) with increased resolution as low as 100 kilobases. With recent technologies, new methods for comprehensive chromosome screening (CCS) like a CGH, qPCR, and single nucleotide polymorphism (SNP) array can detect both euploid and aneuploidy embryos but are unable to detect mosaicism.

Next-generation Sequencing

The DNA sequencing is the process of determining the sequence of nucleotides in a section of DNA.[2-5] The first commercialized method of DNA sequencing was Sanger sequencing. Next-generation sequencing (NGS), also known as high-throughput sequencing, is the term used to describe a number of different modern sequencing technologies. These technologies allow for sequencing of DNA much more quickly and cheaply than the previously used Sanger sequencing and revolutionized the study of genomics and molecular biology. These technologies include:

- *Illumina (Solexa) sequencing:* Illumina sequencing works by simultaneously identifying DNA bases, as each base emits a unique fluorescent signal, and adding them to a nucleic acid chain.
- *Roche 454 sequencing:* This method is based on pyrosequencing, a technique which detects pyrophosphate release, again using fluorescence, after nucleotides are incorporated by polymerase to a new strand of DNA.
- *Ion torrent—Proton/PGM sequencing:* This method of sequencing measures the direct release of H^+ (protons) from the incorporation of individual bases by DNA polymerase and therefore differs from the previous two methods as it does not measure light.

■ PROCESS

The process of PGT includes the steps as described here.

Embryo Biopsy

The embryo biopsy procedure consists of opening the zona pellucida and removal of the cellular material. Zona opening can be performed in three ways:
1. Mechanical:
   a. Direct puncture
   b. Partial zona dissection
2. Chemical (Acid Tyrode's pH = 2.3)
3. Photothermolysis (Laser).

The developmental stages at which biopsy can be performed are as follows:
- *Polar bodies from oocytes (Day 0/Day 1):* 2–3 hours after the ovum pick up, 1st polar body is observed.[6] A small hole of 18–25 μm (not <15 μm) should be made in the zona pellucida with laser or mechanical opening and not to use acid Tyrode here as it can be harmful and could compromise the viability of the oocyte **(Fig. 1)**. Pipettes for polar body biopsy can be beveled or not and the inner diameter should be 12–15 μm.
- *Blastomeres from early cleavage stage embryos (Day 3):* For blastomere biopsy at day 3 of cleavage stage, the blastomere removal is performed in three ways:
   - Blastomere removal by acid Tyrode aspiration **(Fig. 2)**
   - Blastomere removal by extrusion **(Fig. 3)**
   - Blastomere removal by displacement **(Fig. 4)**

It allows the detection of maternal, paternal, and early post-fertilization defects and gives enough time for the genetic diagnosis if it is performed on day 3 and transfer on day 5. Ca^{2+} Mg^{2+} free culture medium facilitates embryo biopsy

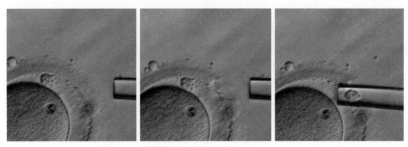

Fig. 1: Polar body biopsy.

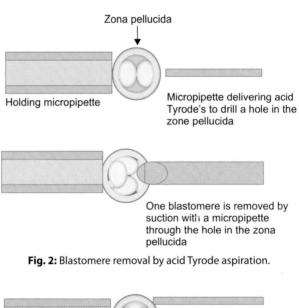

Zona pellucida

Holding micropipette

Micropipette delivering acid Tyrode's to drill a hole in the zone pellucida

One blastomere is removed by suction with a micropipette through the hole in the zona pellucida

Fig. 2: Blastomere removal by acid Tyrode aspiration.

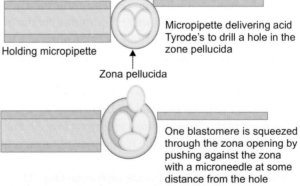

Micropipette delivering acid Tyrode's to drill a hole in the zone pellucida

Holding micropipette

Zona pellucida

One blastomere is squeezed through the zona opening by pushing against the zona with a microneedle at some distance from the hole

Fig. 3: Blastomere removal by extrusion.

with no detrimental effect on embryo development and pregnancy rates (Veiga et al., 1994; Santaló et al., 1996; Dumoulin et al., 1998). Limit exposure time to maximum 10 minutes and after biopsy, gently flush the embryo repeatedly.

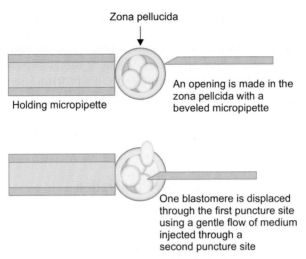

Zona pellucida

Holding micropipette

An opening is made in the zona pellcida with a beveled micropipette

One blastomere is displaced through the first puncture site using a gentle flow of medium injected through a second puncture site

Fig. 4: Blastomere removal by displacement.

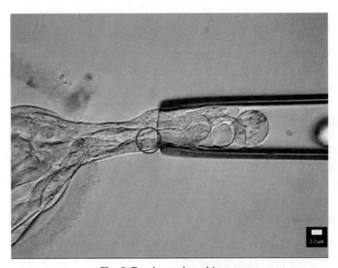

Fig. 5: Trophectoderm biopsy.

- *Trophectoderm cells from blastocysts (Day 5)*: Blastocyst biopsy is an emerging technique as it provides more cells to analyze the defects if present in the embryo.[7-10] It is interesting in monogenic diseases as more DNA is available. A lower degree of mosaicism is observed at this stage and ICM remains fully intact. However, it requires a high blastocyst formation rate, an optimized culture system, and specific laboratory expertise. Genetic results are be obtained in <24 hours in order to avoid cryopreservation **(Fig. 5)**.

Transportation of Biopsied Material to the Genetic Laboratory

The first step in transportation of the sample is proper documentation and form filling with witnessing of the procedure.[2,11] There should be one blank PCR tube for control. The biopsied cells are placed in the PCR tubes with minimum volume of washing media under the stereozoom microscope. The PCR tubes are then placed in the cooler rack, covered with parafilm, and kept inside the shipping box with ice packs. Take care that cooler does not move inside the box during transportation.

Amplification of DNA and Library Preparation

Prepare extraction master mix to extract gDNA and add preamp reagents and incubate for 75 minutes (16 samples), 90 minutes (24 samples), and 150 minutes (96 samples) hands-on time, depending on the panels used. Add barcodes and amp master mix, incubate, pool, purify, and quantitate the library.

Template Preparation

Pipette the library into ion chef cartridge (in case of Ion Torrent) for templating and chip loading. Load the cartridge onto ion chef system. This process takes 15 minutes hands-on time.

Sequencing

Load reagents onto Ion GeneStudio™ S5 systems. Transfer chip onto Ion GeneStudio™ S5 systems for sequencing. This process takes 15 minutes hands-on time.

Analysis

The results are analyzed and interpreted using Torrent Suite™ Software or Ion Reporter™ software **(Figs. 6 and 7)**.

▌ PGT REGULATIONS IN INDIA

In India, Ministry of Family Health and Welfare, regulates the concept under the Pre-conception and Prenatal Diagnostic Techniques (Prohibition of Sex Selection) (PCPNDT) Act, 1994. This is an Act to provide for the prohibition of sex selection, before or after conception, and for regulation of prenatal diagnostic techniques for the purposes of detecting abnormalities or metabolic disorders or chromosomal abnormalities or certain congenital malformations or sex-linked disorders and for the prevention of their misuse for sex determination leading to female feticide.

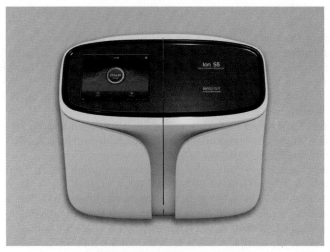

Fig. 6: Ion S5 system Thermo Fisher.

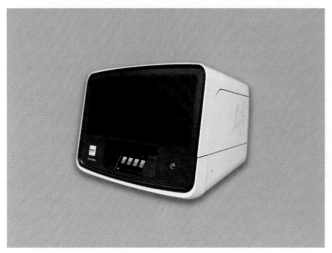

Fig. 7: Ion Chef instrument Thermo Fisher.

Records to be Maintained

Detailed record of the patients that have undergone counseling and tests is to be maintained in the register.

Form D: Form for maintenance of records by the genetic counseling center.

Form E: Maintenance of records by genetic laboratory.

Form F: Form for maintenance of record in case of prenatal diagnostic test/procedure by genetic clinic/ultrasound clinic/imaging center.

Form G: Form of consent (for invasive techniques).

This is in addition to all the consent forms related to IVF procedure as per clinic protocols.

■ REFERENCES

1. Northrop LE, Treff NR, Levy B, Scott Jr RT. SNP microarray-based 24 chromosome aneuploidy screening demonstrates that cleavage-stage FISH poorly predicts aneuploidy in embryos that develop to morphologically normal blastocysts. Mol Hum Reprod. 2010;16(8):590-600.

2. Xuan J, Yu Y, Qing T, Guo L, Shi L. Next-generation sequencing in the clinic: promises and challenges. Cancer Lett. 2013;340(2):284-95.

3. Harton GL, De Rycke M, Fiorentino F, Moutou C, Sengupta S, Traeger-Synodinos J, et al. ESHRE PGD consortium best practice guidelines for amplification-based PGD. Hum Reprod. 2010;26(1):33-40.

4. ACOG Committee Opinion No 430: preimplantation genetic screening for aneuploidy. Obstet Gynecol. 2009;113(3):766-7.

5. Tobler KJ, Ross R, Benner AT, Du L, Brezina PR, Kearns WG. The use of next-generation sequencing (NGS) for preimplantation genetic screening (PGS) and diagnosis (PGD). Fertil Steril. 2014;102(3):e184-5.

6. Verlinsky Y, Ginsberg N, Lifchez A, Valle J, Moise J, Strom CM. Analysis of the first polar body: preconception genetic diagnosis. Hum Reprod. 1990;5(7):826-9.

7. Monk M, Muggleton-Harris AL, Rawlings E, Whittingham DG. Pre-implantation diagnosis of HPRT-deficient male and carrier female mouse embryos by trophectoderm biopsy. Hum Reprod. 1988;3(3):377-81.

8. Franasiak J, Scott RT. (2008). A brief history of preimplantation genetic diagnosis and preimplantation genetic screening. [online] Available from: https://ivf-worldwide.com/cogen/oep/pgd-pgs/history-of-pgd-and-pgs.html [Last accessed January, 2020].

9. Johnson DS, Cinnioglu C, Ross R, Filby A, Gemelos G, Hill M, et al. Comprehensive analysis of karyotypic mosaicism between trophectoderm and inner cell mass. Mol Hum Reprod. 2010;16(12):944-9.

10. Brezina PR, Ross R, Kaufmann R, Anchan R, Zhao Y, Kearns WG. Genetic normalization of differentiating aneuploid cleavage stage embryos. Fertil Steril. 2013;100(3):S69.

11. Harton GL, Magli MC, Lundin K, Montag M, Lemmen J, et al. ESHRE PGD Consortium/Embryology Special Interest Group—best practice guidelines for polar body and embryo biopsy for preimplantation genetic diagnosis/screening (PGD/PGS). Hum Reprod. 2011;26(1):41-6.

9

Ovarian Tissue Cryopreservation

Vineet Mishra

BACKGROUND

Every year, 1,157,294 new cases of cancer get registered in India out of which there are 371,302 cancer-related deaths among females.[1] Although this is a critical health problem, advances in cancer detection and treatment have improved survival rates of female cancer survivors. Most of the alkylating agents and radiation often induce premature failure rendering the woman infertile. Most female cancer patients of reproductive age do not have the option of utilizing established assisted reproductive technologies to safeguard their fertility. In nearly all cancers, with the possible exception of breast cancer, chemotherapy is initiated soon after diagnosis. Because preparation and stimulation for oocyte retrieval usually requires 2–3 weeks or longer, it is generally not feasible to freeze embryos from an adult female cancer patient for potential future use. Even considering the frequent hiatus between surgery and chemotherapy in breast cancer patients, most would not be candidates for oocyte or embryo freezing due to concerns that high estrogen levels might have detrimental effects on the primary tumor. Additionally, not all patients have partners with whom they can create embryos to cryopreserve. Most female cancer patients therefore have limited clinical options for fertility preservation. In select cases, an oophoropexy may be performed to move an ovary out of an intended radiation therapy field. Treatment with gonadotropin-releasing hormone (GnRH) analogs or oral contraceptives during chemotherapy has been advocated to protect the female gonad, although convincing evidence of benefit is yet to be seen. Embryo banking is a proven method but requires both available sperm and several weeks of preparation. Ovarian cryopreservation is a promising clinical technique because it avoids ovarian stimulation and provides the opportunity for preserving gonadal function in prepubertal, as well as adult patients.

OVARIAN CRYOPRESERVATION: A NOVEL OPTION FOR FERTILITY PRESERVATION

There are several methods used to preserve female fertility, including ovarian tissue cryopreservation (OTC) and cryopreservation of embryos and oocytes.

At present, cryopreservation of embryos and oocytes is an accepted clinically established procedure, whereas OTC has not been endorsed by the American Society of Reproductive Medicine and is still considered experimental. Initially, there were only a few case reports. Successful human ovarian transplantation was first reported by Silber et al. with cortical-tissue grafting in monozygotic twins who were discordant for premature ovarian failure.[2] Subsequently, Donnez et al.[3] reported what is deemed to be the first human live birth from orthotropic transplantation of frozen human ovarian tissue in 2004, with another successful live birth achieved by Meirow in 2005.[4] However, it appears now that there is a worldwide live birth rate of over 30–70%, with more than 70 babies.[5] In the opinion of many pioneers, there is now enough evidence to support OTC and to stop considering it an experimental or investigational approach.

Ovarian tissue cryopreservation remains a promising option for female cancer patients who require immediate aggressive gonadotoxic chemotherapy and do not have time for ovarian stimulation and oocyte retrieval. It also remains the only option to preserve fertility among prepubertal girls or women with hormone-sensitive malignancies. In addition, in women undergoing stem cell transplantation for benign hematological diseases (sickle cell disease, aplastic anemia, thalassemia major) and women with autoimmune diseases not responding to immunosuppressive agents, OTC provides a good option to preserve the ovarian tissue. It is also indicated in women carrying genetic mutations for premature ovarian failure. Yet to be mentioned is the growing interest of women in postponing their first pregnancy, owing to education, career planning, or financial instability or even to possible difficulties in finding a partner. Since both the quality and the amount of follicles decrease considerably with age, cryostorage is an alternative for improving pregnancy outcomes.

TECHNIQUES IN OVARIAN TISSUE CRYOPRESERVATION

Ovarian Cortex Tissue

The follicle constitutes the functional unit of the ovary and produces steroids and peptide hormones to regulate the female reproductive cycle. The unique physical distribution of the follicular reserve within the ovary, with the vast majority of small resting follicles located in the outer cortical region and the growing stages of follicles located in the inner medullary region, represents a perfect opportunity to preserve an organ function without freezing the entire organ. By isolating the cortical region, containing 90% of the follicular reserve, human ovarian tissue has been successfully cryopreserved for fertility preservation in young women with cancer diseases for over two decades. Subsequent transplantation of thawed ovarian tissue has restored ovarian endocrine function in 95% of the patients and resulted in the birth of over

130 children worldwide.[6] Ovarian tissue is generally always obtained prior to cancer treatment with the exception of hematological cancers where it is preferable to retrieve tissue after one cycle of chemotherapy. The most common method of tissue retrieval is by laparoscopic method, the other being multiple ovarian tissue biopsies. The superficial cortical tissue must be sharply dissected from the underlying medullary portion of the ovary. The cortex is shaved to a thickness of approximately 1 mm to promote early revascularization once the thawed tissue is transplanted. Once the ovarian tissue is obtained, it is transported on ice and then preserved. This method has historically been associated with ischemia of the cortical tissue after transplantation.

Whole Ovary Cryopreservation

In this method, the whole ovary along with a large vascular pedicle is laparoscopically removed and preserved. If the whole ovary or a large portion is removed, the cortex can be further sectioned into 5 × 5 mm segments and cryopreserved using slow-freeze techniques and vitrification techniques. The long vascular pedicle enables cryoprotectants to reach every cell in the tissue during freezing and vice versa during thawing. It also allows early perfusion of blood from anastomosed vessels and thus reduces early ischemia as seen in ovarian cortical tissue transplantation.[7-8]

■ METHODS OF CRYOPRESERVATION

There are two methods of cryopreservation: (1) slow freezing and (2) vitrification process.

Slow Freezing

This has been the classical method of freezing and uses controlled freezing rates. In any slow freezing process, ice crystals form first outside the cells/tissue. Slow cooling rates allow osmotic adjustments between intra- and extracellular fluid, but they may lead to excessive dehydration and shrinkage. The addition of cryoprotectant agents (CPAs) to the cryopreservation medium helps to overcome these problems. The role of CPAs is to protect the cells against injuries caused by both ice crystals and hypertonicity during cryopreservation. However, CPAs can have osmotic effects upon the cells during freezing/thawing procedures. When cells are exposed to permeating CPAs, they initially undergo dehydration and shrinkage followed by a return to the original volume as the CPA enters the cell. These changes in volume can cause cell damage or even death, depending on their rapidity and magnitude. Addition of CPAs can cause cell damage also by chemical toxicity. Optimal exposure should aim to minimize osmotic stress while avoiding chemical toxicity and allow sufficient permeation and dehydration to achieve protection from freezing injuries.[9]

Cryoprotectant agents are divided into two categories:[10]

1. *Permeating agents*: These are glycerol, dimethyl sulfoxide (DMSO), ethylene glycol, and 1,2-propanediol (PROH); these have a low molecular weight and can pass through the lipid bilayer of the cell membrane, although they do so more slowly than water.

2. *Nonpermeating agents*: These are sugars (sucrose, trehalose, and raffinose) and macromolecules (Ficoll and polyvinylpyrrolidone), as well as proteins and lipoproteins; these remain in the extracellular solution, they are large molecules, and help to promote controlled cell dehydration.

In most slow freezing protocols for ovarian tissue, a combination of one permeating agent and one nonpermeating agent is used. CPA concentrations are around 1.5 M for the permeating agent (usually DMSO) and 0.1 M for the nonpermeating agent (usually sucrose).

Vitrification

Vitrification is a process of converting a supercooled liquid into a glass-like amorphous solid, preventing ice crystal formation. Vitrification processes are based on an ultrafast cooling rate combined with a high concentration of CPAs. However, high concentrations of CPAs have toxic effects on the cells. Because of this, vitrification methods usually use a combination of two or more CPAs, so that the sum of their concentrations supports vitrification, while the low concentration of each CPA reduces their toxic effects.

Cryopreservation by vitrification is attractive because it is a quick and easy procedure and does not require special and expensive equipment. Although it seems simple to perform, if cooling rates are not fast enough, crystallization may occur. In a successful vitrification, the tissue and surrounding solution become transparent, whereas failed vitrification is characterized by an opaque white sample, meaning ice crystals have formed.[11]

Despite the growing popularity of this type of preservation, it is still rarely used for ovarian tissue preservation. Unlike the slow freezing procedure, there is no standard vitrification protocol for ovarian tissue. Apart from the two babies reported by the Japanese group,[11] promising results using vitrified ovarian tissue were also reported by Kiseleva et al.[12] In their case study, vitrified ovarian tissue showed recovery of its reproductive potential after autotransplantation.

▓ THAWING/WARMING AND THE RISK OF RECRYSTALLIZATION

This process is carried out when the frozen ovarian tissue needs to be transplanted or is to be used by the woman. The risk of ice formation during warming is an important factor to be taken into account with slowly frozen or vitrified tissue. Cooling and warming rates interact, and a suitable outcome can be found when both are carefully taken into consideration. The warming

Cryopreservation method	Final CPA concentration	Thawing/warming method
SF	1.5 M EG	10-minute water bath at 37°C; 10-minute baths with lower EG concentrations, sucrose, and PBS at RT
Vitrification	35% EG	TCM 199, SSS, and sucrose at 37°C; 3-minute bath with TCM 199, SSS, and sucrose at RT
SF	1.5 M DMSO	2 minutes in air at RT; water bath at RT; 3 baths in Leibovitz L-15 medium
SF	1.5 M DMSO	30 seconds in air at RT; 2-minute water bath at 37°C; 5-minute baths with lower DMSO concentrations and sucrose

TABLE 1: Examples of thawing/warming protocols described in the literature.

(CPA: cryoprotectant agent; DMSO: dimethyl sulfoxide; EG: ethylene glycol; PBS: phosphate-buffered saline; RT: room temperature; SF: slow freezing; SSS: serum substitute supplement)

procedure of vitrified systems occurs in three phases: (1) conversion of the solution from vitrified into ultraviscous, (2) devitrification (conversion of water into crystalline ice), and (3) recrystallization (growth of very small ice crystals). The formation of small ice nuclei during vitrification is inevitable. However, when sufficient time is available during warming, more nucleation and crystal growth can occur, leading to morphological damage to the tissue. To avoid this, it is essential to increase the warming rate and ensure an adequate CPA concentration.

Once the sample is warmed/thawed, attention should be directed at CPA removal. During this step, an osmotic imbalance may occur due to water uptake suffered by the cells, causing their swelling. This is even worse in vitrified tissue, where higher concentrations of CPAs are present in the tissue fragments. To avoid or minimize this problem, CPA removal can be slowly performed. For this, solutes like proteins (human serum albumin or serum substitute supplement) or sugars (glucose or sucrose) can be used, controlling CPA removal. Usually, a mixture of solutions containing lower CPA concentrations is applied during CPA removal. An overview of some protocols described for human ovarian tissue thawing/warming is shown in **Table 1**.[9]

■ OVARIAN TISSUE TRANSPLANTATION

Given the limited lifespan of ovarian tissue grafts, transplantation should be postponed until the patient is ready to conceive or begins to experience symptoms of ovarian insufficiency. The patient should be in remission from disease, should have support from oncology to proceed with the transplantation and pregnancy, and may benefit from consultation with a perinatologist or high-risk obstetrics specialist to discuss the potential perinatal complications unique to cancer survivors. Ovarian tissue can be transplanted orthotopically to the pelvis or heterotopically to subcutaneous areas such as the forearm or abdomen. Restoration of ovarian function has been reported from both transplantation sites. It appears that peritoneal tissue is superior to subcutaneous tissue as a site of transplantation, likely due to improved revascularization of the transplanted tissue in the peritoneum and subsequent loss of fewer primordial follicles.[13] Transplantation can be performed using laparoscopy or minilaparotomy approaches. Autologous orthotopic transplantation of previously frozen cortical tissue has led to a series of live births and is currently the most effective technique for transplantation.

Although OTC is a promising option for fertility preservation, it is associated with certain ethical concerns regarding duration of graft, reseeding of malignant cells, embryo and oocyte quality, risks associated with surgery for retrieval and reimplantation, and reproductive outcomes following transplantation.

■ CONCLUSION

Ovarian tissue cryopreservation prior to cancer treatment and subsequent transplantation after cancer is an exciting, yet investigational, option for fertility preservation. A multidisciplinary team of experts including oncologists and reproductive endocrinologists will best achieve this assessment. Although the impact of specific cancer treatment regimens on ovarian function may be uncertain, patients should be given reasonable estimates of risk with the best available evidence as they make informed decisions about undertaking investigational procedures to preserve their fertility and/or restore hormonal function.

■ REFERENCES

1. National Cancer Registry Statistics, India.
2. Silber SJ, Lenahan KM, Levine DJ, Pineda JA, Gorman KS, Friez MJ, et al. Ovarian transplantation between monozygotic twins discordant for premature ovarian failure. N Engl J Med. 2005;353:58-63.
3. Donnez J, Dolmans MM, Demylle D, Jadoul P, Pirard C, Squifflet J, et al. Livebirth after orthotopic transplantation of cryopreserved ovarian tissue. Lancet. 2004;364:1405-10.
4. Meirow D, Levron J, Eldar-Geva T, Hardan I, Fridman E, Zalel Y, et al. Pregnancy after transplantation of cryopreserved ovarian tissue in a patient with ovarian failure after chemotherapy. N Engl J Med. 2005;353:318-21.
5. Silber S. Ovarian tissue cryopreservation and transplantation: scientific implications. J Assist Reprod Genet. 2016;33:1595-603.
6. Kristensen SG, Andersen CY. OTC—more than just fertility preservation. 2018;9:1-2.
7. Oktem O, Oktay K. A novel ovarian xenografting model to characterize the impact of chemotherapy agent on human primordial follicle reserve. Cancer Res. 2007;67 (21):10159-62.

8. Practice Committee of American Society for Reproductive Medicine; Practice Committee of Society for Assisted Reproductive Technology. Ovarian tissue and oocyte cryopreservation. Fertil Steril. 2008;90:S241-6.

9. Rivas Leonel EC, Lucci CM, Amorim CA. Cryopreservation of human ovarian tissue: a review. Transfus Med Hemother. 2019;46(3):173-81.

10. Amorim CA, Curaba M, Van Langendonckt A, Dolmans MM, Donnez J. Vitrification as an alternative means of cryopreserving ovarian tissue. Reprod Biomed Online. 2011;23(2):160-86.

11. Suzuki N, Yoshioka N, Takae S, Sugishita Y, Tamura M, Hashimoto S, et al. Successful fertility preservation following ovarian tissue vitrification in patients with primary ovarian insufficiency. Hum Reprod. 2015;30(3):608-15.

12. Kiseleva M, Malinova I, Komarova E, Shvedova T, Chudakov K. The Russian experience of autotransplantation of vitrified ovarian tissue to a cancer patient. Gynecol Endocrinol. 2014;30(Suppl 1):30-1.

13. Kondapalli LA. Ovarian tissue cryopreservation and transplantation. In: Gracia C, Woodruff TK (Eds). Oncofertility Medical Practice: Clinical Issues and Implementation, illustrated edition. New York: Springer Science & Business Media; 2012. pp. 63-76.

10 Laparoscopic Cervicopexy

Aswath Kumar, Chaithra TM, Sandip Datta Roy

▦ INTRODUCTION

Pelvic organ prolapse (POP) is a common problem. Around one in two women above 50 years of age have this condition. A wide variety of treatment options are available for the treatment of POP, including conservative approaches and surgical techniques. POP surgeries can be done via vaginal, laparotomy, and laparoscopic approaches. In this chapter, we will be discussing uterus-sparing laparoscopic cervicopexy. Laparoscopic approach offers a good panoramic view of the pelvic anatomy; thus, a one-sitting approach (global approach) for treating the POP and associated disorders is possible via the same surgical route. Its advantages over other techniques include better surgical exposure, less pain, shorter hospital stay, and fewer recurrences.[1]

However, for a variety of reasons such as preservation of female identity (psychological) and functional preservation (sexual, bowel, and bladder), many women may desire uterine preservation rather than hysterectomy. Over the years, various treatment options for POP for women who desire uterine conservation have been described, such as the vaginal Fothergill procedure, transvaginal uterosacral suspension, sacrospinous fixation of vault or uterus, sacrocervicopexy, pectineal ligament suspension, retropubic suspension, or round ligament suspension.[2] They are associated with high recurrence rates.

▦ APICAL PROLAPSE: UTERINE DESCENT/VAULT PROLAPSE

DeLancey level 1 support which is provided by the cardinal and uterosacral ligament complex[3] forms the apical support for the uterus and upper vagina. Its disruption may result in uterine or vaginal vault prolapse. In addition to apical prolapse, they are associated with cystocele, urethrocele, stress urinary incontinence, and recurrences.[4-6] Many studies have shown that the anterior vaginal wall is the site of recurrences.[4,6]

▦ CURRENT TREATMENTS FOR PELVIC ORGAN PROLAPSE (NICE–GUIDELINES 2018)

The guidelines suggest to treat only symptomatic prolapses. Nonsevere POP Q1 and 2 may be treated with conservative measures such as pelvic floor muscle training, electrical stimulation, and biofeedback. We can even try vaginal estrogen therapy and pessaries conservatively. Severe form of POP Q3 and 4 attracts surgical procedures.[7]

Traditionally, vaginal hysterectomy with pelvic floor native tissue repair or Manchester repair was practiced, both with high recurrence rates. Now more uterine preserving approaches are stressed upon due to enumerate reasons such as preservation of female identity, sexuality, and bowel and bladder function. In this chapter, we are covering different laparoscopic cervicopexy techniques and their benefits.

Relative contraindications to uterine preservation during prolapse surgery are malignancy, complex hyperplasia, severe endometriosis, dysfunctional uterine bleeding, chronic pelvic pain, and large uterine myomas. All of these conditions need discussion with patients seeking uterine conservation. Postcervicopexy mesh procedures and hysterectomy are more challenging.

■ LAPAROSCOPIC SACROCERVICOPEXY

First performed in 1992 by Lane abdominally, later in 2007 by Nezhat laparoscopically, laparoscopic sacrocervicopexy has now been accepted all over the world as gold standard procedure.

Principle

Nonabsorbable soft polypropylene mesh is fixed to pubovesical fascia and rectovaginal fascia to sacral promontory using nonabsorbable sutures or tackers. Salient anatomical landmarks for this procedure are sacral promontory dissection keeping right ureter and pelvic vessels in mind, medial to right ureter and lateral to right uterosacral ligament till the rectovaginal fascia **(Figs. 1A to D)**.

First, the presacral space dissection is performed keeping salient landmarks in mind **(Fig. 1A)** with clearance of the fibrofatty tissue covering the promontory, keeping a good plane of dissection to avoid bleeding (from the left common iliac vein and sacral vessels). Next, the peritoneum is lifted up and dissected using harmonic shears or monopolar hook, toward the right uterosacral ligament medial to the right ureter. Polypropylene monofilament mesh is usually interposed between the vagina and the bladder anteriorly and the rectum posteriorly **(Fig. 1B)**. The Y-shaped mesh is fixed, anteriorly over the anterior vaginal wall at the level of the bladder trigone and posteriorly over the puborectalis muscle and rectovaginal fascia over the upper vagina. In subtotal hysterectomy, both meshes are sutured using nonabsorbable suture together at the level of the isthmus, and then only one limb of the mesh is fixed to the anterior longitudinal ligament at the level of S1/S2 **(Fig. 1C)**. According to preoperative discussion, subtotal hysterectomy is performed wherever necessary.

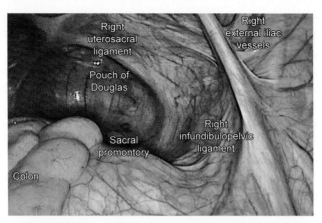

Fig. 1A: Salient anatomical landmarks for sacrocervicopexy.

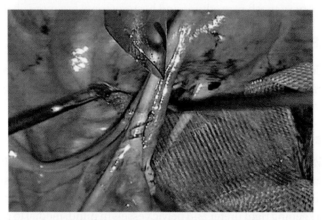

Fig. 1B: Polypropylene monofilament meshes being interposed between the vagina and the bladder anteriorly and the rectum posteriorly.

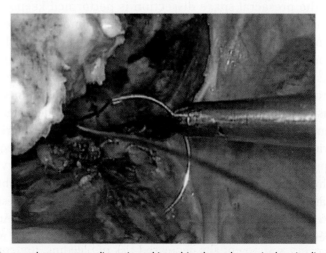

Fig. 1C: After sacral promontory dissection taking a bite through anterior longitudinal ligament.

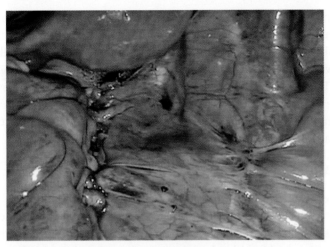

Fig. 1D: Complete peritonization of the mesh at the end of the procedure.
(*Courtesy*: Dr Sushila Saini)

TABLE 1: Complications of sacrocervicopexy.			
Complications	*Incidence*	*Prevention*	*Management*
• Mesh-related • Bowel herniation	1%	• Use soft macroporous polypropylene mesh • Bacterial infection • Devascularization • (The in situ cervix acts as a barrier to bacterial infection from vagina and maintains vascularization)	• Low threshold for re-exploration • Complete repertorization of mesh[8]
Mesh erosion[9,10]	• 3% • With concomitant hysterectomy, the complication is 10–14%	• Prevent suture exposure vaginally • Avoid total hysterectomy along with sacrocolpopexy/ sacrocervicopexy	
Spondylodiscitis			Laparotomy/ laparoscopic removal of mesh
Vertebral abscess[11]		Prevent mesh exposure vaginally	Complete mesh excision

Complications of Sacrocervicopexy

The complications of sacrocervicopexy are given in **Table 1**.

The laparoscopic hysteropexy (laparoscopic hysteropexy vs. concomitant hysterectomy with sacrocolpopexy) has potential advantages of a relatively quick recovery and potentially decreased risk of bleeding, ureteral injury, adhesion formation, and mesh extrusion vaginally.[10,12,13] So some authors recommend hysteropexy over concomitant hysterectomy.[14-17] This procedure also enables the vaginal length to be maintained and provides substantial subjective improvement in prolapse symptoms, sexual function, and quality of life.[10] The risk of developing a uterine malignancy is only 0.6%,[18] especially in those who preferred to preserve the uterus. In addition, malignant transformation of myomas is extremely rare (0.1–0.3%).[19] There are limited data regarding subsequent pregnancy after this type of procedure.

■ LAPAROSCOPIC PECTOPEXY

Pectopexy is an alternative to sacrocervicopexy or colpopexy. It is a mesh-augmented site-specific repair, in which anterior support pubocervical fascia is attached to iliopectineal ligament (prolongation of the Cooper's ligament) on both sides. It should be done by experienced and trained laparoscopic surgeons. It is also applicable for vault prolapse and after subtotal hysterectomy for vault suspension.[20]

Pectopexy Technique

For pectopexy, we follow the procedure as described by Noé.[21] The peritoneal layer is first opened along the right round ligament toward the pelvic side wall. Then an incision in the medial and caudal direction is made with a Harmonic scalpel, and the right external iliac vein is identified **(Fig. 2A)**. Fatty tissue in this area is dissected with Harmonic scalpel and a small segment of the right iliopectineal ligament (Cooper's ligament) adjacent to the insertion of the iliopsoas muscle is exposed **(Fig. 2B)**. One should be careful about the

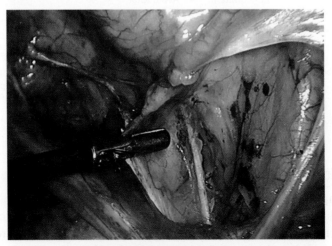

Fig. 2A: Right external iliac vein.

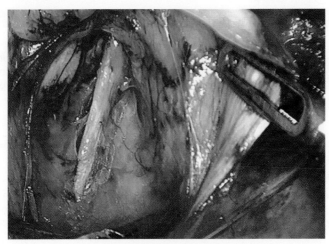

Fig. 2B: Left iliopectineal ligament.
(*Courtesy*: Dr Sushila Saini)

obturator nerve which lies medially and also about the presence of circumflex iliac vein just above the pectineal ligament.

The same procedure is then repeated on the left side of the patient. In patients with an intact uterus, the anterior peritoneum over the cervix is dissected down for mesh fixation. After completion of dissection, a 3 × 15 cm long strip of soft polypropylene mesh is introduced into the abdominal cavity through a 10-mm trocar and the ends of the mesh are sutured to both iliopectineal ligaments by intracorporeal suturing using Ethibond or Prolene No. 1-0 sutures. The mesh is also fixed over the anterior aspect of the cervix with Ethibond suture in a tension-free manner. Finally, the peritoneum over the mesh is sutured with No. 1 vicryl suture.

Current evidence on the safety and efficacy of laparoscopic mesh pectopexy for apical prolapse of the uterus or vagina is insufficient in quality and quantity. Therefore, this procedure should only be used in the context of research by trained surgeons.[7]

PECTOPEXY VERSUS SACROCERVICOPEXY

The differences between pectopexy and sacrocervicopexy are given in **Table 2**.

LAPAROSCOPIC MODIFIED KHANNA'S SLING PROCEDURE

Laparoscopic Khanna's sling surgery is laparovaginal procedure wherein the uterine prolapse is corrected by fixing a Mersilene tape to the posterior aspect of cervix and the anterior superior iliac spine (ASIS). We have modified the procedure by using a soft polypropylene mesh (30 × 3 cm) instead of tape. Application of mesh gives a better and stronger hold on the cervix.

TABLE 2: Pectopexy versus sacrocervicopexy.

	Sacrocervicopexy	Pectopexy
Technique	Tape is fixed from fixed points on pericervical ring to anterior longitudinal ligament at L5-S1 junction passing through rectovaginal space to right pararectal region	Bilateral tape is fixed from fixed points on pericervical ring to pectineal ligament—organ-free area
Synthetic mesh being used	Soft polypropylene (most commonly 15 × 3 cm Y-shaped)	Soft polypropylene (most commonly—T-shaped)
Peritonization	Needed	Needed
Narrow pelvic space for surgery, especially in obese	Present	No narrow spaces (wide area in the pelvis, allows surgeons to react more satisfactorily in complex surgical conditions[22])
Damage to rectum	Chances are high	Very unlikely
Damage to hypogastric plexus	Near promontory dissection+	Nil
De novo SUI	7–50%	Less likely
Defecation disorders	17–34%	Nil
Dangerous complication	Mesh erosion	Iliac vein injury

(SUI: stress urinary incontinence)

The procedure begins by making a transverse incision on the posterior cervicovaginal junction and separating the vaginal wall from the cervix. The pouch of Douglas (POD) is opened. The midpoint of a 30 × 3 cm mesh is fixed on the posterior aspect of the cervix with No. 1-0 Prolene. The two ends of the mesh are pushed inside the POD and the posterior vaginal incision is closed with No. 2-0 vicryl **(Figs. 3A to F)**.

A small incision is made 1 cm medial and superior to the ASIS and a long laparoscopic needle holder is introduced through the incision and passed between the two layers of the broad ligament. The needle holder is brought out through the posterior cervical incision and the ends of the mesh are pulled out on both sides. The uterine prolapse is corrected by pulling and adjusting the mesh. The ends of the mesh are fixed to the inguinal ligament close to the ASIS with No. 1 Prolene. This is a simple procedure and can be easily replicated. In our unpublished series of more than 100 cases, we have not encountered any mesh erosion, infection, and vascular or ureteric injuries **(Figs. 3G to N)**.

Laparoscopic cervicopexy is a promising uterine procedure with other advantages of improved visualization of pelvic anatomy, shorter hospitalization, less postoperative pain, and a quicker return to normal activities.

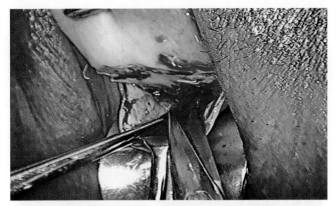

Fig. 3A: Pouch of Douglas opened using scissors.

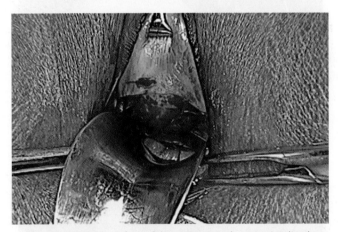

Fig. 3B: Posterior surface of the supravaginal cervix visualized.

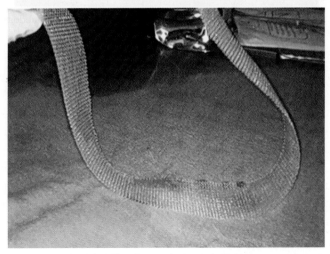

Fig. 3C: Soft polypropylene mesh 30 × 3 cm.

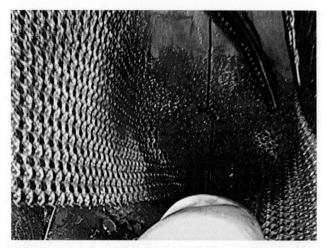

Fig. 3D: Center of the mesh anchored to posterior cervix using Prolene.

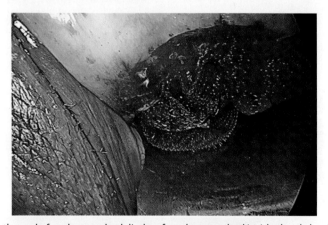

Fig. 3E: At the end of anchorage, both limbs of mesh are pushed inside the abdominal cavity.

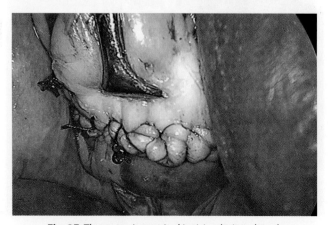

Fig. 3F: The posterior vaginal incision being closed.

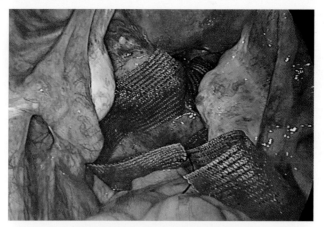

Fig. 3G: Laparoscopic view of mesh.

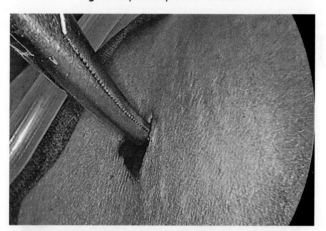

Fig. 3H: A small incision above and medial to anterior superior iliac spine.

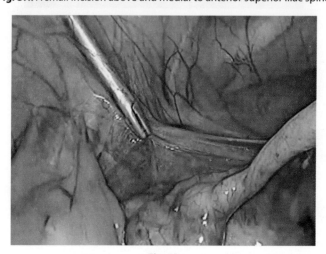

Fig. 3I

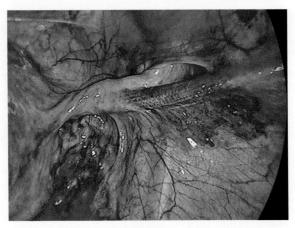

Fig. 3J

Figs. 3I and J: Peritoneum over the round ligament is lifted to facilitate entry of needle holder along the round ligament through the skin incision medial to anterior superior iliac spine to reach posterior aspect of the cervix.

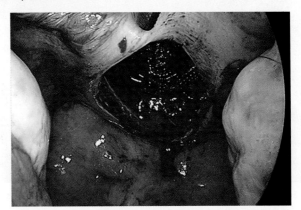

Fig. 3K: Mesh is adjusted by pulling both sides out of the skin incisions till the prolapse is corrected.

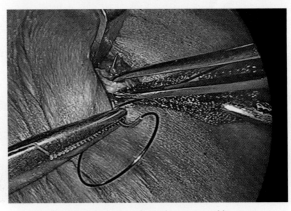

Fig. 3L: Mesh being anchored to inguinal ligament.

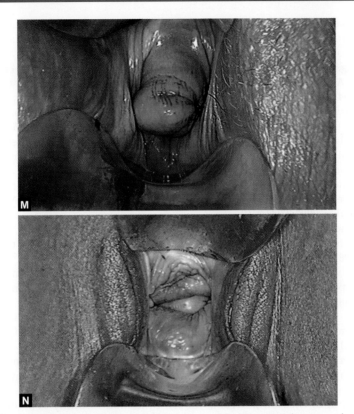

Figs. 3M and N: Prolapse after correction by modified Khanna's sling procedure.

REFERENCES

1. Khunda A, Vashisht A, Cutner A. New procedures for uterine prolapse. Best Pract Res Clin Obstet Gynaecol. 2013;27(3):363-79.
2. Diwan A, Rardin CR, Kohli N. Uterine preservation during surgery for uterovaginal prolapse: a review. Int Urogynecol J Pelvic Floor Dysfunct. 2004;15(4):286-92.
3. DeLancey JO. Anatomic aspects of vaginal eversion after hysterectomy. Am J Obstet Gynecol. 1992;166(6 Pt 1):1717-24.
4. Summers A, Winkel LA, Hussain HK, DeLancey JO. The relationship between anterior and apical compartment support. Am J Obstet Gynecol. 2006;194(5):1438-43.
5. Hendrix SL, Clark A, Nygaard I, Aragaki A, Barnabei V, McTiernan A. Pelvic organ prolapse in Women's Health Initiative: gravity and gravidity. Am J Obstet Gynecol. 2002;186(6):1160-6.
6. Fialkow MF, Newton KM, Weiss NS. Incidence of recurrent pelvic organ prolapse 10 years following primary surgical management: a retrospective cohort study. Int Urogynecol J Pelvic Floor Dysfunct. 2008;19(11):1483-7.
7. National Institute for Health and Care Excellence (NICE). Laparoscopic mesh pectopexy for apical prolapse of the uterus or vagina. Published March 14, 2018.
8. Trompoukis P, Nassif J, Gabriel B, Wattiez A. Internal hernia after laparoscopic sacrocervicopexy. J Minim Invasive Gynecol. 2011;18(4):525-7.

9. Serati M, Bogani G, Sorice P, Braga A, Torella M, Salvatore S, et al. Robot-assisted sacrocolpopexy for pelvic organ prolapse: a systematic review and meta-analysis of comparative studies. Eur Urol. 2014;66(2):303-18.

10. Nygaard IE, McCreery R, Brubaker L, Connolly A, Cundiff G, Weber AM, et al. Abdominal sacrocolpopexy: a comprehensive review. Obstet Gynecol. 2004;104(4):805-23.

11. Downing KT. Vertebral osteomyelitis and epidural abscess after laparoscopic uterus-preserving cervicosacropexy. J Minim Invasive Gynecol. 2008;15(3):370-2.

12. Culligan PJ, Blackwell L, Goldsmith LJ, Graham CA, Rogers A, Heit MH. A randomized controlled trial comparing fascia lata and synthetic mesh for sacral colpopexy. Obstet Gynecol. 2005;106(1):29-37.

13. Maher C, Baessler K, Glazener CM, Adams EJ, Hagen S. Surgical management of pelvic organ prolapse in women: a short version Cochrane review. Neurourol Urodyn. 2007;27(1):3-12.

14. Cundiff GW, Varner E, Visco AG, Zyczynski HM, Nager CW, Norton PA, et al. Risk factors for mesh/suture erosion following sacral colpopexy. Am J Obstet Gynecol. 2008;199(6):688.e1-5.

15. Bensinger G, Lind L, Lesser M, Guess M, Winkler HA. Abdominal sacral suspensions: analysis of complications using permanent mesh. Am J Obstet Gynecol. 2005;193(6):2094-8.

16. Tan-Kim J, Menefee S, Luber K, Nager C, Lukacz E. Prevalence and risk factors for mesh erosion after laparoscopic-assisted sacrocolpopexy. Int Urogynecol J. 2011;22(2):205-12.

17. Cvach K, Geoffrion R, Cundiff GW. Abdominal sacral hysteropexy: a pilot study comparing sacral hysteropexy to sacral colpopexy with hysterectomy. Female Pelvic Med Reconstr Surg. 2012;18(5):286-90.

18. Ramm O, Gleason J, Segal S, Antosh D, Kenton K. Utility of preoperative endometrial assessment in asymptomatic women undergoing hysterectomy for pelvic floor dysfunction. Int Urogynecol J. 2012;23(7):913-7.

19. Wallach EE, Vlahos NF. Uterine myomas: an overview of development, clinical features, and management. Obstet Gynecol. 2004;104(2):393-406.

20. Rivoire C, Botchorishvili R, Canis M, Jardon K, Rabischong B, Wattiez A, et al. Complete laparoscopic treatment of genital prolapse with meshes including vaginal promontofixation and anterior repair: A series of 138 patients. J Minim Invasive Gynecol. 2007;14(6):712-8.

21. Noé KG, Schiermeier S, Alkatout I, Anapolski M. Laparoscopic pectopexy: a prospective, randomized, comparative clinical trial of standard laparoscopic sacral colpocervicopexy with the new laparoscopic pectopexy-postoperative results and intermediate-term follow-up in a pilot study. J Endourol. 2015;29(2):210-5.

22. Kale A, Biler A, Terzi H, Usta T, Kale E. Laparoscopic pectopexy: initial experience of single center with a new technique for apical prolapse surgery. Int Braz J Urol. 2017;43(5):903-9.

11 Screening for Breast Cancer

Karishma Kirti, Nita S Nair ■

■ INTRODUCTION

Breast cancer is the most common cancer among women worldwide. In 2018, 1,62,468 new cases were reported in India, making it the most common cancer in females (27.7%). It is also the leading cause of cancer death responsible for 11.1% of all cancer deaths in 2018.[1] The incidence of breast cancer is increasing with a significant urban to rural divide.[2]

Screening is defined as the identification of an unrecognized disease in an apparently healthy, asymptomatic population by means of tests, examinations or other procedures that can be applied rapidly and easily to the target population.

Accuracy of a screening test is based on its ability to distinguish disease from nondisease.

Biases are also of concern in relation to screening namely, lead time, length time, and selection bias **(Table 1 and Fig. 1)**. One of the most alarming consequences of screening is overdiagnosis which leads to significant anxiety and burdens the healthcare system.

■ SCREENING IN BREAST CANCER

Screening for breast cancer has over the years become synonymous to the use of mammography (MMG) alone. However, the role of physical examination or

TABLE 1: Biases associated with screening.

Lead time bias	Increased survival is a function of the time gained before the point at which the disease would have become evident in the absence of screening although the time of death remains the same **(Fig. 1A)**
Length time bias	The tendency to detect slow growing tumors as more aggressive tumors are like to present as interval cancers **(Fig. 1B)**
Selection bias	It is the tendency for individuals who are health conscious to participate in screening trials
Overdiagnosis bias	Diagnosis of a disease that could have potentially not been diagnosed throughout life with death due to another cause eventually

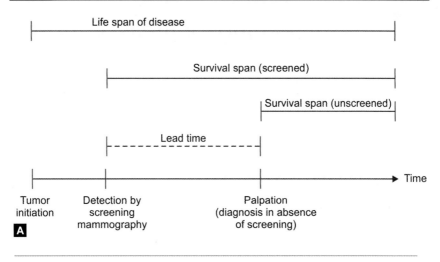

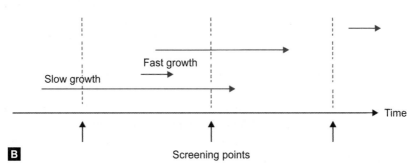

Figs. 1A and B: (A) Lead time bias; (B) Length bias.

clinical breast examination (CBE) by trained healthcare professionals needs to be given due consideration. Ideally, a screening tool for breast cancer should reduce mortality from breast cancer and also all-cause mortality, have a low false positive rate, and be inexpensive **(Box 1)**.

- Breast self-examination (BSE)
- Clinical breast examination (CBE)
- Screening by imaging—MMG/USG/MRI

■ AVAILABLE MODALITIES FOR SCREENING

Breast Self-examination

Because of its simplicity and low cost, breast self-examination (BSE) appears to be the most appropriate method for early breast cancer screening. However, there are no studies that show its effect on reducing mortality. There are two landmark trials that evaluated the role of BSE as a screening tool.

> **BOX 1:** Principles of screening.
>
> The effectiveness of any screening is measured by various means:
> *Disease requirements:*
> - Disease must be serious in nature with significant rates of morbidity and/or mortality
> - Effective treatment should be available
> - Natural history should be well understood to identify the window of opportunity for early detection and effective treatment or possibly a cure
> - Disease must not be too rare
>
> *Screening test requirements:*
> - Easy and inexpensive
> - Safe and acceptable to individuals as well as physicians
> - Reproducible
> - Level of accuracy should be adequate
>
> *Healthcare system requirements:*
> Follow-up care should be available for all who test positive

- *Shanghai trial:*[3] This trial included 266,064 factory workers in Shanghai. Women were randomized into BSE instruction group versus not. The tumor size, stage, and cumulative breast cancer mortality rate were not significantly different between the two groups. The study concluded that intensive instruction in BSE cannot reduce mortality rate of breast cancer, but more and smaller benign breast lumps can be detected.
- *Russian trial:*[4] This study of 122,471 women from St Petersburg randomized women to BSE versus not. Final results showed no difference in mortality, though the BSE group had higher 15-year survival rates (53.2% vs. 45.8%, $p = 0.051$). The indications for biopsy were more than double in the experimental arm (7.5% vs. 3.5%, $p <0.01$).
- *A meta-analysis* conducted by *Hackshaw et al.*[5] which included these two randomized controlled trials (RCTs) and 20 observational studies also concluded that BSE is not an effective method of reducing breast cancer mortality. The success of BSE depends on the subject's motivation and her recognition of breast cancer as a real threat to her. Studies have shown poor attendance at breast teaching classes and low compliance with monthly breast examination. Nevertheless, it increases awareness about breast cancer and breast health.

Clinical Breast Examination

The role of MMG as a screening tool has been criticized over the years. Sensitivity of MMG in a premenopausal population is low, and efficacy as a screening tool has been debatable. In women above 50 years of age, MMG by itself as well as in combination with CBE has shown a reduction in cause-specific mortality. Unfortunately, it also led to approximately 25% overdiagnosis after 25 years of follow-up.[6] A change to CBE may reduce the detection of indolent invasive as well as noninvasive cancers and may reduce overdiagnosis.

There are three RCTs that directly evaluate the role of CBE for breast cancer:

1. *The Philippines study*:[7] In 1995, *Pisani et al.* randomized women aged 35–64 years to five annual clinical examinations of the breasts (carried out by trained nurses/midwives) versus not. The first round of examinations included 151,168 women, who were also instructed in the technique of BSE and provided with a leaflet in the local language explaining the purpose and methodology of BSE. Because of the poor compliance with follow-up of screen positive women, even with home visits, the active intervention was discontinued after completion of the first screening round in December 1997.

2. *The Trivandrum study*:[8] *Sankarnarayanan et al.* initiated a study in the Trivandrum district in 2006 wherein they randomized 1,15,652 healthy women, aged 30–69 years, to intervention (CBE) or control (no screening). The percentage of early-stage (stage IIA or lower) breast cancer in the intervention versus control groups was 43.8% versus 25.4% ($p = 0.023$), while advanced-stage (stage IIB or higher) breast cancer was 45.0% versus 68.3% ($p = 0.005$). Thus, suggesting that there was a downstaging of cancers noted in the CBE arm.

3. *The Mumbai study*:[9] This study, started in 1998 by *Mittra et al.,* randomized 151,538 women into intervention group (CBE by healthcare workers + 2 yearly monitoring) and control group (Health education at entry). After three rounds of screening, they noted a significant downstaging in breast cancer in the screening arm ($p = 0.004$) **(Tables 2 to 4)**. The results of its impact on mortality are awaited.

TABLE 2: Staging at diagnosis (breast-screening arm).

Monitoring rounds	Early stage (0 + I + II)	Late stage (III+ IV)	Staging not available	Total
One	21 (70.00%)	9 (30.00%)	2	32
Interval cancers	17 (73.91%)	6 (26.09%)	4	27
Two	15 (68.18%)	7 (31.82%)	2	24
Interval cancers	13 (92.86%)	1 (7.14%)	3	17
Three	12 (57.14%)	9 (42.86%)	4	25

TABLE 3: Staging of asymptomatic referrals at diagnosis (breast-control arm).

Monitoring rounds	Early stage (0 + I + II)	Late stage (III+ IV)	Staging not available	Total
One	2 (66.67%)	1 (33.33%)	0	3
Two	18 (54.55%)	15 (45.45%)	6	39
Three	18 (46.15%)	21 (53.85%)	6	45

Study	Cancers detected in screened population	Interval cancers	CBE		Down staging	
			Sensitivity	Specificity	Screened	Control
Mumbai study	73	37	57.44%	91.99%	Early lesions 78 Advanced 38	Early lesion 32 Advanced lesion 37
Philippines study	68	NA	53.2%	100%	17% more advanced cases in control group	
Trivandrum Study	80	28	54.1%	94%	Early lesion 43.8% Advanced lesion 45.0%	Early lesion 25.4% Advanced lesions 68.3%

TABLE 4: Efficacy of randomized controlled studies for combined modality breast cancer screening (MMG and CBE).

Imaging Modalities

Mammography

There are several RCTs evaluating the role of screening MMG in breast cancer **(Table 5)**:

- *The Health Insurance Plan (HIP) study*[10] was the first RCT which was designed to show the role of screening in mortality reduction in breast cancer, using MMG and CBE (by trained surgeons). 6,200 women aged 40-64 years were included in the study. The results after 18 years of recruitment reported a relative risk (RR) for death from breast cancer to be 0.77 (0.52–1.13) for women aged 40–49, 0.79 (0.58–1.08) for women aged 50–64, and an overall RR of 0.78 (0.61–1.00).

- *The Edinburgh Randomized Trial of Breast Cancer Screening*[11] recruited 44,288 women aged 45–64 years during 1978–81. A total of 22,944 women were randomized into the study group and were offered screening for 7 years; the remaining women formed the control group. After 10 years, breast cancer mortality was 14–21% lower in the study group than in the controls (not statistically significant).

- *Canadian National Breast Screening Study (CNBSS) I and II:*[12] This is the only randomized study that answers the question of contribution of MMG over and above CBE. Nearly 90,000 women were randomized in the CNBSS studies.

TABLE 5: Screening details of the randomized trials of breast cancer screening using mammography.

Study	Year	Age at entry (In years)	Numbers screened		Screening interval and rounds of screening 5 rounds	Available follow-up
			Screened	Control	Mammography + CBE vs. CBE/not and number of rounds of screening	
HIP	1963–1969	40–64	31,000	31,000	Annual MMG + CBE vs. Not 3 rounds	18 years
Edinburgh	1978–1991	45–64	22,944	21,344	2 yearly MMG + annual CBE (7 rounds)	10 years
CNBSS I	1980	40–49	44,925	44,910	Annual MMG + CBE + BSE vs. One time CBE + BSE at initial evaluation	25 years
CNBSS II	1980	50–59			Annual MMG + CBE + BSE vs. Annual CBE + BSE	25 years
UK Age trial	1990–1997	39–48	53,883	106,953	Annual MMG	17 years
Malmo I	1976–1978	45–70	21,088	21,195	MMG every 18–24 months (5 rounds)	30 years
Malmo II	1978–1990	43–49	9,587	8,199	MMG every 18–24 months	22 years
Swedish two county trial	1977–1979	40–74	77,080	55,985	40–49 years: MMG every 2 years 50–74 years: MMG every 3 years	29 years
Stockholm trial	1981–1985	40–64	40318	20000	MMG every 2 years (2 rounds)	25 years
Göteborg trial	1982–1991	39–59	21,650	29,961	MMG every 18 months (5 rounds)	25 years

The CNBSS 1 randomized 50,489 women aged 40–49 years old to MMG + CBE versus usual health care. At the end of 16-year follow-up, there was no significant difference in breast cancer mortality between the two groups.

The CNBSS II included women aged 50–59 years and randomized them to annual MMG + CBE + BSE to annual CBE + BSE alone to determine how much breast cancer mortality was reduced by the addition of MMG.

The MMG + CBE + BSE detected more node-negative and small breast cancers than screening with CBE + BSE alone. However, this had no impact on breast cancer mortality. The risk of a false positive result was 49.1% (95% CI 40.3–64.1) after 10 MMG and 22.3% (95% CI 19.2–27.5) after 10 CBEs.[13]

At 25 years of follow-up,[13] of the 666 cancers detected in the MMG arm during the screening period, 454 cancers detected in the MMG arm and 524 in the control arm were palpable tumors.

There was one over-diagnosed breast cancer for every 424 women who received MMG screening in the trial. Overall, 1,005 women died from breast cancer during the 25-year follow-up period (1.1%). The 25-year cumulative mortality from all causes of death and breast cancer specific mortality was similar between the MMG and control arms (1.02, 0.98–1.06; $p = 0.28$) and (0.99, 0.88–1.12; $p = 0.87$), respectively.

- *UK Age trial:*[14] 160,921 women 40–48 years were randomized to a ratio of 1:2 to an intervention group of annual MMG and control group of usual medical care. A significant reduction in breast cancer mortality was noted in the intervention group compared with the control group in the first 10 years after diagnosis (RR 0·75, 0·58–0·97) but not thereafter (RR 1·02, 0·80–1·30) from tumors diagnosed during the intervention phase. The overall breast cancer incidence during 17-year follow-up was similar between the intervention group and the control group (RR 0·98, 0·93–1·04).

- *The Malmo trial:*[15] This study randomized birth year cohorts into screening versus not. Overall, women in the study group aged greater than or equal to 55 had a 20% reduction in mortality from breast cancer [35 vs. 44; relative risk 0.79 (0.51–1.24)]. A more recent related study[16] assessed the rate of over diagnosis in the screening group at the end of 15 years and found it to be 10% in the 55–69 year group.

- *Swedish Two-County trial:*[17] A total of 133,065 women aged 40–74 years residing in two Swedish counties (Dalarna and Östergötland) were randomized into a group invited to mammographic screening and a control group receiving usual care. There was a significant reduction in breast cancer mortality in women invited to screening according to both local end point committee data (RR = 0.69; 95% CI: 0.56–0.84; p <0.0001) and consensus data (RR = 0.73; 95% CI: 0.59–0.89; $p = 0.002$). At 29 years of follow-up, the number of women needed to undergo screening for 7 years to prevent one breast cancer death was 414 according to local data and 519 according to consensus data.

- *Stockholm mammographic screening trial:*[18] 40,318 women from 40 to 64 years of age were randomized into single view MMG for two screening rounds versus no intervention. Overall, after a mean follow-up of 11.2 years, a nonsignificant mortality reduction of 26% was seen. In women aged 40–49 years, there was no effect on mortality was found whereas in the 50–64 years age group, a 38% mortality reduction was observed which was significant.
- *Göteborg breast screening trial:*[19] This trial randomized 51,611 women aged 39–49 years to MMG screening every 18 months. They found a nonsignificant 21% reduction in mortality from breast carcinoma (RR 0.79, $p = 0.14$) by Endpoint Committee (EPC model) and a borderline significant, 23% rate reduction was observed using the SCB follow-up model (RR 0.77, $p = 0.05$).

Cochrane review:[20,21] This landmark review carried out by Olsen and Gøtzsche, classified the trials into two groups—adequately randomized and inadequately randomized.

Adequately randomized	Suboptimally randomized
Malmo I trial	New York HIP trial
Canadian trial	Malmo II trial
UK age trial	Swedish 2 county trial
	Göteborg trial
	Stockholm trial
	Edinburgh trial—not included

If only adequately randomized trials were looked at, there was no reduction in 7- or 13-year breast cancer mortality (RR 0.90, CI 0.79–1.02). However, when only inadequately randomized trials were included, both 7- and 13-year reduction in breast cancer mortality were decreased significantly (RR 0.75). The RR for all seven trials was 0.81.

They concluded that breast cancer mortality is an unreliable outcome and biased in the favor of screening and although the studies were underpowered to assess all-cause mortality, there was no benefit in all-cause mortality with screening MMG in any age group irrespective of the kind of trial (adequately/inadequately randomized trial).

In conclusion, they noted that for every 2,000 women invited for screening throughout 10 years, one will avoid dying of breast cancer and 10 healthy women, who would not have been diagnosed if there had not been screening, will be treated unnecessarily.

Ultrasound

A combination of MMG and ultrasound (USG) for screening of breast cancer has shown increased detection rate (improved sensitivity) which comes

TABLE 6: ACR BI-RADS categories, 5th edition.

		Likelihood of cancer
Category 0	Incomplete—additional imaging needed	N/A
Category 1	Negative	Essentially 0%
Category 2	Benign	Essentially 0%
Category 3	Probably benign	0 to≤2%
Category 4 4a: 4b: 4c:	Suspicious Low suspicion of malignancy Moderate suspicion of malignancy High suspicion of malignancy	 >2 to ≤10% >10 to ≤50% >50 to <95%
Category 5	Highly suggestive of malignancy	≥95%
Category 6	Known biopsy—proven malignancy	N/A

(ACR: American College of Radiology; BI-RADS: Breast Imaging Reporting and Data System)

at a cost of unacceptable high-false positives and increased biopsy rates. Adding a single screening USG to MMG in women with elevated risk of breast cancer will yield an additional 1.1–7.2 cancers per 1,000 high-risk women, but it will also substantially increase the number of false positives.[22] However, there is no study that shows reduction in mortality due to incremental value of USG to MMG. It can at best serve as an additional tool to MMG screening in women with intermediate risk for breast cancer (personal history of breast cancer or biopsies associated with increased risk or relative with early onset breast cancer). The final assessment of USG lesions is also categorized by BI-RADS scoring **(Table 6)**.

Magnetic Resonance Imaging

Magnetic resonance imaging (MRI) has proven to be more sensitive than MRI for patients with higher than average risk for breast cancer. It is universally recommended for women who are BRCA1 or BRCA2 positive and for women higher than 25% lifetime risk of breast cancer. A German study[23] assessed MRI for supplemental screening for women with average risk of breast cancer (lifetime risk <15%) and found that MRI helped identify additional breast cancers that were not detected with MMG or USG with an additional cancer yield of 15.5 per 1,000 cases. The additional cancers diagnosed were small (median size 8 mm), mostly node negative (93%) and tended to exhibit adverse biological profile. The interval cancer rate was 0%. They suggested the used of MR raging as supplemental tool in average risk women, especially those with dense breasts.

▦ EFFECTIVENESS OF SCREENING

Downstaging

The aim of screening interventions is to detect the disease in the early stages and allow timely intervention and treatment. Most screening studies have demonstrated increased incidence in the screened arm compared to control arm with no difference in mortality. However, the lesions picked up in the screened arm are early breast cancers. Only if the intervention can conclusively demonstrate downstaging of breast cancer, can it be expected to impact breast cancer-related mortality.

Overdiagnosis

Overdiagnosed lesions refer to disease that would never have become clinically apparent without screening before a patient's death. In an overview of seven autopsy studies, the median prevalence of occult invasive breast cancer was 1.3% (range 0–1.8%) and of ductal carcinoma in situ was 8.9% (range, 0–14.7%).[24,25] Treatment of these cancers would constitute overtreatment.

Overdiagnosis is a prominent flaw with the use of MMG and CBE may offer respite to the same. Kalager et al.[6] pointed out that the amount of overdiagnosis observed in the previous RCTs is strikingly similar (22–24%). The concern with overdiagnosis is clinicians cannot identify which impalpable lesions detected by screening MMG will never progress within the lifetime of the women and thus have to treat all diagnosed lesions.

It may be argued that much of the overdiagnosis that occurs with MMG may be avoided by CBE alone. As the sensitivity of CBE is low, there is a possibility of false negative findings. However, since the specificity of CBE is high, false positivity rates are low.

Adverse Effects

While the efficacy and effectiveness of breast cancer screening have been proven by randomized studies, little attention is paid to the side effects of screening which are mainly due to false positive screen findings, necessitating further diagnostic imaging and biopsy rates. The psychological anxiety of a false positive finding as well as the morbidity of additional testing is also often ignored.

Cost-effectiveness

Determining the cost-effectiveness of CBE alone is difficult because no completed trial has really compared CBE versus no screening. Sarvazyan et al. reviewed the diagnostic accuracy, cost, and cost-effectiveness of breast cancer screening strategies worldwide. They concluded that in view of many countries with limited resources, more affordable strategies like CBE have the potential for providing effective screening for breast cancer.

	ACR	ACS	ACOG	NCCN	USPSTF	ACP
Age to start MMG	40	45 with option to start at 40	Offer at 40, no later than 50	40	50	50 with shared decision at 40
Age to stop MMG	No age limit: Tailor to individual health status	When life expectancy is <10 years	Age 75, then shared decision	Not stated	74	74, or in women life expectancy <10 years
MMG interval	Annual	Annual 45–54; annual/biennial in 55 and older	Annual or biennial	Annual	Biennial	Biennial

■ CONCLUSION

- Awareness and breast self-examination as a tool for awareness in woman of all ages
- No role of screening mammogram in women <50 years
- No screening recommendations for premenopausal women, only awareness to breast cancer
- Annual clinical breast examination and awareness about breast cancer or biennial MMG in healthy women over the age of 50 years
- However, the 25% probability of overdiagnosis must be kept in mind when recommending MMG as a screening tool. The additional biopsy need for a facility for localization for impalpable lesions, related anxiety, and referral to cancer centers need to be considered when advising a screening mammogram
- High-risk individuals (BRCA positive, significant family history) to be treated as per standard guidelines
- *Breast self-examination*: No evidence of reduction in mortality; useful as an awareness tool
- *Clinical breast examination*: No published data on reduction mortality; effective in downstaging
- *Imaging*: Reduction in mortality in women over the age of 50 years; associated with 25% overdiagnosis; no mortality reduction in women <50 years of age

■ REFERENCES

1. Bray F, Ferlay J, Soerjomataram I, Siegel RL, Torre LA, Jemal A. Global Cancer Statistics 2018: GLOBOCAN estimates of incidence and mortality worldwide for 36 cancers in 185 countries. CA Cancer J Clin. 2018;68(6):394-424.

2. Nagrani RT, Budukh A, Koyande S, Panse NS, Mhatre SS, Badwe R. Rural urban differences in breast cancer in India. Indian J Cancer. 2014;51(3):277-81.

3. Thomas DB, Gao DL, Ray RM, Wang WW, Allison CJ, Chen FL, et al. Randomized trial of breast self-examination in Shanghai: final results. J Natl Cancer Inst. 2002;94(19):1445-57.

4. Semiglazov VF, Manikhas AG, Moiseenko VM, Protsenko SA, Kharikova RS, Seleznev IK, et al. Results of a prospective randomised investigation [Russia(St. Petersburg)/WHO] to evaluate the significance of self-examination for the early detection of breast cancer. Vopr Onkol. 2003;49(4):434-41.

5. Hackshaw AK, Paul EA. Breast self-examination and death from breast cancer: a meta-analysis. Br J Cancer. 2003;88(7):1047-53.

6. Kalager M, Adami HO, Bretthauer M, Tamimi RM. Overdiagnosis of invasive breast cancer due to mammography screening: results from the Norwegian screening program. Ann Intern Med. 2012;156(7):491-9.

7. Pisani P, Parkin DM, Ngelangel C, Esteban D, Gibson L, Munson M, et al. Outcome of screening by clinical examination of the breast in a trial in the Philippines. Int J Cancer. 2006;118(1):149-54.

8. Sankaranarayanan R, Ramadas K, Thara S, Muwonge R, Prabhakar J, Augustine P, et al. Clinical breast examination: preliminary results form a cluster randomised controlled trial in India. J Natl Cancer Inst. 2011;103(19):1476-80.

9. Mittra I, Mishra GA, Singh S, Aranke S, Notani P, Badwe R, et al. A cluster randomized, controlled trial of breast and cervix cancer screening in Mumbai, India: methodology and interval results after three rounds of screening. Int J Cancer. 2010;126(4):976-84.

10. Shapiro S, Strax P, Venet L. Periodic breast cancer screening in reducing mortality from breast cancer. JAMA. 1971;215(11):1777-85.

11. Alexander FE. The Edinburgh Randomised trial of breast cancer screening. J Natl Cancer Inst Monogr. 1997;1997(22):31-5.

12. Miller AB, Baines CJ, To T, Wall C. Canadian National breast Screening Study: 2. Breast cancer detection in death rates among women aged 50 to 59 years. CMAJ. 1992;147(10):1477-88.

13. Miller AB, Wall C, Baines CJ, Sun P, To T, Narod SA. Twenty five year follow up for breast cancer incidence and mortality of the Canadian Nation Breast Cancer Screening Study: randomised screening trial. BMJ. 2014;348:g366.

14. Moss SM, Wale C, Smith R, Evans A, Cuckle H, Duffy SW. Effect of mammographic screening from age 40 years on breast cancer mortality in the UK Age Trial at 17 years' follow-up: a randomised controlled trial. Lancet Oncol. 2015;16(9):1123-32.

15. Andersson I, Aspegren K, Janzon L, Landberg T, Lindholm K, Linell F, et al. Mammographic screening and mortality from breast cancer: the Malmö mammographic screening trial. BMJ. 1988;297(6654):943-8.

16. Zackrisson S, Andersson I, Manjer J, Garne JP. Rate of over-diagnosis of breast cancer 15 years after end of Malmö mammographic screening trial: follow-up study. BMJ. 2006;332(7543):689-92.

17. Tabár L, Vitak B, Chen TH, Yen AM, Cohen A, Tot T, et al. Swedish two-county trial: Impact of mammographic screening on breast cancer mortality during 3 decades. Radiology. 2011;260(3):658-63.

18. Frisell J, Lidbrink E, Hellström L, Rutqvist L-E. Follow-up after 11 years - update of mortality results in the Stockholm mammography screening trial. Breast Cancer Res Treat. 1997;45(3):263-70.

19. Bjurstam N, Björneld L, Warwick J, Sala E, Duffy SW, Nyström L, et al. The Gothenburg breast screening trial. Cancer. 1997;80(11):2091-9.

20. Olsen O, Gøtzsche PC. Cochrane review on screening for breast cancer with mammography. Lancet. 2001;358(9290):1340-2.

21. Gøtzsche PC, Jørgensen KL. Screening for breast cancer with mammography. Cochrane Database Syst Rev. 2013;(6):CD001877.

22. Berg WA, Blume JD, Cormack JB, Mendelson EB, Lehrer D, Böhm-Vélez M, et al. Combined screening with ultrasound and mammography vs mammography alone in women at elevated risk of breast cancer. JAMA. 2008;299(18):2151-63.

23. Kuhl CK, Strobel K, Bieling H, Leutner C, Schild HH, Schrading S. Supplemental breast MR imaging screening of women with average risk of breast cancer. Radiology. 2017;283(2):361-70.

24. Welch HG, Black WC. Using autopsy series to estimate the disease "reservoir" for ductal carcinoma in situ of the breast: how much more breast cancer can we find? Ann Intern Med. 1997;127(11):1023-8.

25. Black WC, Welch HG. Advances in diagnostic imaging and overestimations of disease prevalence and the benefits of therapy. N Engl J Med. 1993;328(17): 1237-43.

Index

Page numbers followed by *f* refer to figure, *fc* refer to flowchart, and *t* refer to table